Intracardiac Echo Imaging in Atrial and Ventricular Arrhythmia Ablation

Editors

PASQUALE SANTANGELI
FERMIN C. GARCIA
LUIS C. SÁENZ

CARDIAC ELECTROPHYSIOLOGY CLINICS

www.cardiacEP.theclinics.com

Consulting Editors
RANJAN K. THAKUR
ANDREA NATALE

June 2021 • Volume 13 • Number 2

ELSEVIER

1600 John F. Kennedy Boulevard • Suite 1800 • Philadelphia, Pennsylvania, 19103-2899

http://www.theclinics.com

CARDIAC ELECTROPHYSIOLOGY CLINICS Volume 13, Number 2
June 2021 ISSN 1877-9182, ISBN-13: 978-0-323-79626-2

Editor: Joanna Collett
Developmental Editor: Arlene Campos

Cardiac Electrophysiology Clinics (ISSN 1877-9182) is published quarterly by Elsevier Inc., 360 Park Avenue South, New York, NY 10010-1710. Months of issue are March, June, September, and December. Subscription prices are $238.00 per year for US individuals, $502.00 per year for US institutions, $249.00 per year for Canadian individuals, $535.00 per year for Canadian institutions, $303.00 per year for international individuals, $535.00 per year for international institutions and $100.00 per year for US, Canadian and international students/residents. To receive student/resident rate, orders must be accompanied by name of affiliated institution, date of term, and the signature of program/residency coordinator on institution letterhead. Orders will be billed at individual rate until proof of status is received. Foreign air speed delivery is included in all Clinics subscription prices. All prices are subject to change without notice. **POSTMASTER:** Send address changes to Cardiac Electrophysiology Clinics, Elsevier Health Sciences Division, Subscription Customer Service, 3251 Riverport Lane, Maryland Heights, MO 63043. **Customer Service: 1-800-654-2452 (US and Canada). From outside of the US and Canada, call 314-477-8871. Fax: 314-447-8029. E-mail: JournalsCustomerService-usa@elsevier.com (for print support); JournalsOnlineSupport-usa@elsevier.com (for online support).**

Reprints. For copies of 100 or more of articles in this publication, please contact the Commercial Reprints Department, Elsevier Inc., 360 Park Avenue South, New York, NY 10010-1710. Tel.: 212-633-3874; Fax: 212-633-3820; E-mail: reprints@elsevier.com.

Cardiac Electrophysiology Clinics is covered in *MEDLINE/PubMed (Index Medicus)*.

Contributors

CONSULTING EDITORS

RANJAN K. THAKUR, MD, MPH, MBA, FHRS
Professor of Medicine and Director, Arrhythmia
Service, Thoracic and Cardiovascular Institute,
Sparrow Health System, Michigan State
University, Lansing, Michigan

ANDREA NATALE, MD, FACC, FHRS
Executive Medical Director of the Texas
Cardiac Arrhythmia Institute, St. David's
Medical Center, Professor, Dell Medical

School, University of Texas at Austin, Austin,
Texas; National Medical Director, Cardiac
Electrophysiology, Consulting Professor,
Division of Cardiology, Stanford University,
Stanford, California; Clinical Professor of
Medicine, Case Western Reserve University,
Cleveland, Ohio; Director, Interventional
Electrophysiology, Scripps Clinic, San Diego,
California

EDITORS

PASQUALE SANTANGELI, MD, PhD
Associate Professor of Medicine,
Electrophysiology Section, Cardiovascular
Division, Hospital of the University of
Pennsylvania, Philadelphia, Pennsylvania, USA

FERMIN C. GARCIA, MD
Associate Professor of Medicine,
Electrophysiology Section, Cardiovascular

Division, Hospital of the University of
Pennsylvania, Philadelphia, Pennsylvania, USA

LUIS C. SÁENZ, MD
Cardiac Electrophysiologist, Director Cardiac
Electrophysiology, Fundacion CardioInfantil,
Bogota, Colombia

AUTHORS

AMIN AL-AHMAD, MD
Texas Cardiac Arrhythmia Institute, St. David's
Medical Center, Austin, Texas, USA

MAHESH BALAKRISHNAN, MBBS
Division of Cardiovascular Medicine, University
of Arizona College of Medicine Tucson,
Tucson, Arizona, USA

CHRISTOPHER BARRETT, MD, FACC
Division of Cardiology, Section of Cardiac
Electrophysiology, University of Colorado
School of Medicine Anschutz Medical
Campus, Aurora, Colorado, USA

MARCO BERGONTI, MD
Heart Rhythm Center, Centro Cardiologico
Monzino IRCCS, Milan, Italy

JASON S. BRADFIELD, MD
UCLA Cardiac Arrhythmia Center, David
Geffen School of Medicine at UCLA, Los
Angeles, California, USA

J. DAVID BURKHARDT, MD
Texas Cardiac Arrhythmia Institute, St. David's
Medical Center, Austin, Texas, USA

TIMOTHY CAMPBELL, BSc
Department of Cardiology, Westmead
Hospital; Westmead Applied Research Centre,
University of Sydney, Sydney, New South
Wales, Australia

MICHELA CASELLA, MD, PhD
Cardiology and Arrhythmology Clinic,
University Hospital "Ospedali Riuniti",
Department of Clinical, Special and Dental

Sciences, Marche Polytechnic University,
Ancona, Italy

PAOLO COMPAGNUCCI, MD
Cardiology and Arrhythmology Clinic,
University Hospital "Ospedali Riuniti",
Department of Biomedical Sciences and Public
Health, Marche Polytechnic University,
Ancona, Italy

ANDRE D'AVILA, MD, PhD
Beth Israel Deaconess Medical Center,
Boston, Massachusetts, USA

DOMENICO G. DELLA ROCCA, MD
Texas Cardiac Arrhythmia Institute, St. David's
Medical Center, Austin, Texas, USA

LUIGI DI BIASE, MD
Texas Cardiac Arrhythmia Institute, St.
David's Medical Center, Austin, TX, USA;
Montefiore Medical Center, Bronx, New York,
USA

TIMM MICHAEL DICKFELD, MD, PhD
Professor of Medicine and Cardiac
Electrophysiologist, Section of Cardiac
Electrophysiology, Maryland Arrhythmia and
Cardiac Imaging Group (MACIG), University of
Maryland School of Medicine, Baltimore,
Maryland, USA

ANDRES ENRIQUEZ, MD
Division of Cardiology, Queen's University,
Kingston, Ontario, Canada

CAROLA GIANNI, MD
Texas Cardiac Arrhythmia Institute, St.
David's Medical Center, Austin, Texas,
USA

MATTHEW HANSON, MD
Division of Cardiology, Queen's University,
Kingston, Ontario, Canada

HARIS HAQQANI, MD, PhD
Associate Professor, Prince Charles Hospital,
University of Queensland, Brisbane,
Queensland, Australia

JANA HASKOVA, MD
Department of Cardiology, Institute for Clinical
and Experimental Medicine, Prague, Czech
Republic

RODNEY P. HORTON, MD
Texas Cardiac Arrhythmia Institute, St. David's
Medical Center, Austin, Texas, USA

**MATHEW D. HUTCHINSON, MD, FACC,
FHRS**
Professor of Medicine, Division of
Cardiovascular Medicine, University of Arizona
College of Medicine Tucson, Tucson, Arizona,
USA

JOSEF KAUTZNER, MD, PhD
Department of Cardiology, Institute for Clinical
and Experimental Medicine, Prague, Czech
Republic; Palacky University Medical School,
Olomouc, Czech Republic

HOUMAN KHAKPOUR, MD
UCLA Cardiac Arrhythmia Center, David
Geffen School of Medicine at UCLA, Los
Angeles, California, USA

SAURABH KUMAR, BSc(Med), MBBS, PhD
Associate Professor, Department of
Cardiology, Westmead Hospital; Westmead
Applied Research Centre, University of
Sydney, Sydney, New South Wales,
Australia

FRANTISEK LEHAR, MD, PhD
Department of Cardiology, Institute for Clinical
and Experimental Medicine, Prague;
Department of Internal Medicine 1–
Cardioangiology, St Anne's University
Hospital, Brno, Czech Republic

SHUMPEI MORI, MD, PhD
UCLA Cardiac Arrhythmia Center, David
Geffen School of Medicine at UCLA, Los
Angeles, California, USA

ANDREA NATALE, MD, FACC, FHRS
Executive Medical Director of the Texas
Cardiac Arrhythmia Institute, St. David's
Medical Center, Professor, Dell Medical
School, University of Texas at Austin, Austin,
Texas; National Medical Director, Cardiac
Electrophysiology, Consulting Professor,
Division of Cardiology, Stanford University,
Stanford, California; Clinical Professor of
Medicine, Case Western Reserve University,
Cleveland, Ohio; Director, Interventional
Electrophysiology, Scripps Clinic, San Diego,
California

NICHOLAS PALMERI, MD
Beth Israel Deaconess Medical Center,
Boston, Massachusetts, USA

APOOR PATEL, MD
Division of Cardiac Electrophysiology,
Department of Cardiology, Houston
Methodist DeBakey Heart and Vascular
Center, Houston Methodist Hospital,
Houston, Texas, USA

RAJEEV KUMAR PATHAK, MBBS, PhD
Associate Professor of Cardiology, Clinical
Lead of Cardiac Electrophysiology Unit,
Department of Cardiology, Australian National
University, Canberra Hospital, Canberra,
Australian Capital Territory, Australia

PIERRE C. QIAN, MBBS, PhD
Department of Cardiology, Westmead
Hospital, Sydney, Australia

DEEP CHANDH RAJA, MBBS, MD
Clinical Cardiac Electrophysiology Fellow,
Department of Cardiology, Australian
National University and Canberra hospital,
Canberra, Australian Capital Territory,
Australia

ALEJANDRO JIMENEZ RESTREPO, MD
Cardiac Electrophysiologist, Section of
Cardiology, Marshfield Clinic Health System,
Marshfield, Wisconsin, USA

ANTONIO DELLO RUSSO, MD, PhD
Cardiology and Arrhythmology Clinic,
University Hospital "Ospedali Riuniti",
Department of Biomedical Sciences and Public
Health, Marche Polytechnic University,
Ancona, Italy

EDUARDO B. SAAD, MD, PhD
Cardiac Arrhythmia and Pacing, Center for
Atrial Fibrillation - Hospital Pró-Cardíaco and
Hospital Samaritano Botafogo, Rio de Janeiro,
Brazil

MOUHANNAD M. SADEK, MD
Arrhythmia Service, Division of Cardiology,
Department of Medicine, The Ottawa Hospital,
Ottawa, Ontario, Canada

JAVIER E. SANCHEZ, MD
Texas Cardiac Arrhythmia Institute, St. David's
Medical Center, Austin, Texas, USA

PRASHANTHAN SANDERS, MBBS, PhD
Professor of Cardiology, Director of Centre for
Heart Rhythm Disorders, University of Adelaide
and Royal Adelaide Hospital, Adelaide,
Australia

ROBERT D. SCHALLER, DO
Electrophysiology Section, Division of
Cardiovascular Medicine, Perelman School of
Medicine at the University of Pennsylvania,
Philadelphia, Pennsylvania, USA

KALYANAM SHIVKUMAR, MD, PhD
UCLA Cardiac Arrhythmia Center, David
Geffen School of Medicine at UCLA, Los
Angeles, California, USA

USHA B. TEDROW, MD, MS
Cardiovascular Division, Department of
Medicine, Brigham and Women's Hospital,
Boston, Massachusetts, USA

CLAUDIO TONDO, MD, PhD, FESC
Heart Rhythm Center, Centro Cardiologico
Monzino IRCCS; Department of Clinical
Sciences and Community Health, University of
Milan, Milan, Italy

WENDY S. TZOU, MD, FACC, FHRS
Associate Professor of Medicine, Director
of Cardiac Electrophysiology, Division of
Cardiology, Section of Cardiac
Electrophysiology, University of
Colorado School of Medicine Anschutz
Medical Campus, Aurora, Colorado,
USA

MIGUEL VALDERRÁBANO, MD
Division of Cardiac Electrophysiology,
Department of Cardiology, Houston
Methodist DeBakey Heart and Vascular
Center, Houston Methodist Hospital,
Houston, Texas, USA

Contents

cardiac anatomy, ICE is used to guide electrophysiology procedures and monitor for complications. This article is a short overview of the application of real-time ICE imaging during atrial fibrillation ablation procedures.

Left atrial appendage closure (LAAC) is an increasingly common procedure for patients with nonvalvular atrial fibrillation and contraindications to long-term anticoagulation. Traditionally, LAAC has been performed under transesophageal echocardiography (TEE) guidance. Although most operators have become experienced and comfortable with TEE-guided appendage closure, there has been a growing interest in the use of intracardiac echocardiography (ICE) for LAAC. This article describes the rationale and technique for ICE-guided LAAC.

Catheter ablation is the most effective treatment option for idiopathic ventricular arrhythmias. Intracardiac echocardiography (ICE) has been increasingly used during ablation procedures, allowing real-time visualization of cardiac anatomy, and improving our understanding of the relationships between different cardiac structures. In this article we review the adjuvant role of ICE to guide mapping and ablation of ventricular arrhythmias in the structurally normal heart.

 Video content accompanies this article at http://www.cardiacep.theclinics.com.

Intracardiac echocardiography (ICE) is a valuable tool in cardiac ablation procedures, especially in ablation of ventricular arrhythmias. The article details how ICE can aid in ablation of ventricular arrhythmias in nonischemic cardiomyopathy.

Catheter ablation of arrhythmias in congenital heart disease can be a challenging undertaking with often complicated anatomic considerations. Understanding this anatomy and the prior surgical repairs is key to procedural planning and a successful outcome. Intracardiac echocardiography (ICE) adds complimentary real-time visualization of anatomy and catheter positioning along with other imaging modalities. In addition, ICE can visualize suture lines, baffles, and conduits from repaired congenital heart disease and forms a useful part of the toolkit required to deal with these complex arrhythmias.

Video content accompanies this article at http://www.cardiacep.theclinics.com.

The effective diagnosis and management of procedural complications remains an important challenge for electrophysiology operators. Intracardiac echocardiography provides a real-time imaging modality with spectral and color Doppler capabilities that integrates directly with electroanatomic mapping systems. It provides detailed characterization of anatomic variants, which allows the operator to optimize the ablation strategy to the individual thereby avoiding the inherent risk of excessive or ineffective lesions. Complications, such as intracardiac thrombus or pericardial effusion, can be detected and managed before the onset of clinical symptoms. Intracardiac echocardiography facilitates the diagnosis and management of intraoperative hypotension.

 Video content accompanies this article at http://www.cardiacep.theclinics.com.

This article reviews the basis for image integration of intracardiac echocardiography (ICE) with three-dimensional electroanatomic mapping systems and preprocedural cardiac imaging modalities to enhance anatomic understanding and improve guidance for atrial and ventricular ablation procedures. It discusses the technical aspects of ICE-based integration and the clinical evidence for its use. In addition, it presents the current technical limitations and future directions for this technology. This article also includes figures and videos of clinical representative arrhythmia cases where the use of ICE is key to a safe and successful outcome.

 Video content accompanies this article at http://www.cardiacep.theclinics.com.

Interest in endomyocardial biopsy (EMB) has progressively grown during the past decade. Still, its use remains limited to highly specialized centers, mostly because it is considered an invasive procedure with poor diagnostic yield and inherent complications. Indeed, the diagnostic performance of EMB is strictly linked to the sample of myocardium we can obtain. If we can precisely localize areas of diseased myocardium, sampling error or inadequate withdrawals are minimized. In this state-of-the-art review, we provide guidance on how to technically and practically perform EMB guided by electroanatomic voltage mapping and intracardiac echocardiography, and review the evidence supporting this combined approach.

 Video content accompanies this article at http://www.cardiacep.theclinics.com.

Catheter-based ultrasonography is a widely used tool in cardiac electrophysiology practice, and intracardiac echocardiography is supplanting other forms of imaging to become the dominant imaging modality. Given advances in pericardial access, intrapericardial echocardiography can be performed using ultrasound catheters as well. Intrapericardial echocardiography and echocardiography from the coronary sinus, also an epicardial structure, allows interventionalists to obtain unique views from virtually any vantage point, compared with other forms of echocardiography. Both intrapericardial echocardiography and coronary sinus echocardiography are safe and important alternatives that can be used during complex procedures in the electrophysiology laboratory.

 Video content accompanies this article at http://www.cardiacep.theclinics.com.

Intracardiac echocardiography (ICE) is the most practical method for online imaging during electrophysiological procedures. It allows guiding of complex catheter ablation procedures together with electroanatomical mapping systems, either with minimal or with zero fluoroscopy exposure. Besides safe and reproducible transseptal puncture, ICE helps to assess location and contact of the tip of the ablation catheter relative to specific anatomical structures. Another option is visualization of the arrhythmogenic substrate in patients with ventricular arrhythmias. This article describes the clinical utility of ICE in non-fluoroscopic electrophysiology procedures more in detail.

 Video content accompanies this article at http://www.cardiacep.theclinics.com.

Transvenous lead extraction is an invaluable procedure within the contemporary management of cardiac implantable electronic devices. Transvenous lead extraction has traditionally been guided by fluoroscopy. Complementary imaging with intracardiac echocardiography can provide valuable additional information, such as identification of complications, lead-adherent echodensities, and sites of lead-tissue adherence. As such, it can be used to aid in risk stratification before lead removal, help to choose tools or techniques, and provide visual monitoring throughout the procedure. Intracardiac echocardiography can be incorporated into the lead extraction workflow of the contemporary electrophysiologist and provide valuable information supporting safety and efficacy.

With real-time three-dimensional ultrasound, live volumetric images with adequate spatial and temporal resolution are obtained to accurately display structures with complex anatomy and guide interventional procedures. In this review, we will provide an overview of current ultrasound technologies that allow for real-time three-dimensional imaging, with a focus on their application for three-dimensional intracardiac echocardiography.

CARDIAC ELECTROPHYSIOLOGY CLINICS

SERIES OF RELATED INTEREST

Cardiology Clinics
Available at: https://www.cardiology.theclinics.com/
Heart Failure Clinics
Available at: https://www.heartfailure.theclinics.com/
Interventional Cardiology Clinics
Available at: https://www.interventional.theclinics.com/

THE CLINICS ARE AVAILABLE ONLINE!
Access your subscription at:
www.theclinics.com

Foreword
Intracardiac Echocardiography

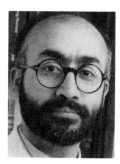 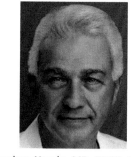

Ranjan K. Thakur, MD, MPH, MBA, FHRS   Andrea Natale, MD, FACC, FHRS

Consulting Editors

We are pleased to introduce the readers to the current issue of the *Cardiac Electrophysiology Clinics* on "Intracardiac Echo Imaging in Atrial and Ventricular Arrhythmia Ablation," edited by Drs Garcia, Saenz, and Santangeli.

Echocardiography is an integral part of cardiology. The first catheter-mounted ultrasound transducer was introduced in 1960, but the introduction of lower-frequency catheters (<12 MHz) in the 1990s made intracardiac imaging widely applicable. Initially, radial intracardiac echocardiography (ICE) was most useful for vascular procedures, and later, for transseptal catheterization, but the availability of phased-array intracardiac ultrasound catheters opened up applications in electrophysiology.

The most impressive impact of ICE has been on aiding anatomic visualization of the fossa ovalis during transseptal catheterization. This has allowed rapid dissemination of safe transseptal catheterization globally, even in the hands of novices, and allowed atrial fibrillation ablation to become widely utilized.

This issue of the *Cardiac Electrophysiology Clinics* discusses the use of ICE for definition of normal cardiac anatomy as well as transseptal catheterization, ablation of atrial and ventricular arrhythmias, closure of the left atrial appendage, early recognition of procedural complications, and other emerging innovative uses.

We thank the editors and all the contributors for summarizing the applications of a very important tool in electrophysiology. We hope the readership will find these articles useful as summaries to review current utility of ICE in clinical electrophysiology.

Ranjan K. Thakur, MD, MPH, MBA, FHRS
Sparrow Thoracic and Cardiovascular Institute
Michigan State University
1440 East Michigan Avenue; Suite 400
Lansing, MI 48912, USA

Andrea Natale, MD, FACC, FHRS
Texas Cardiac Arrhythmia Institute
Center for Atrial Fibrillation at
St. David's Medical Center
1015 East 32nd Street, Suite 516
Austin, TX 78705, USA

E-mail addresses:
thakur@msu.edu (R.K. Thakur)
andrea.natale@stdavids.com (A. Natale)

Card Electrophysiol Clin 13 (2021) xiii
https://doi.org/10.1016/j.ccep.2021.04.001
1877-9182/21/© 2021 Published by Elsevier Inc.

Preface

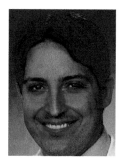
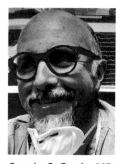
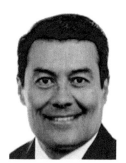

Pasquale Santangeli, MD, PhD   Fermin C. Garcia, MD   Luis C. Sáenz, MD

Editors

The introduction of intracardiac echocardiography (ICE) undoubtedly represents a major advancement in cardiac imaging, and it has become an integral part of a variety of percutaneous interventional and electrophysiology procedures. ICE allows for real-time assessment of cardiac anatomy, can guide catheter manipulation in relation to the different anatomic structures, and provides invaluable monitoring for potential complications, such as thrombus formation or pericardial effusion. The uniqueness of ICE compared with other intraprocedural imaging modalities, such as transesophageal echocardiography, is that it can be performed by the primary operator and under conscious sedation, without the need for general anesthesia. In addition, ICE has helped to reduce fluoroscopy exposure to both the patient and the operator, with a potential beneficial effect on total procedure time and outcomes. This issue is entirely focused on the utility of ICE for the invasive electrophysiology procedure and aims to provide the readers with a comprehensive, state-of-the-art review of the utility of ICE by international leaders in the field. Each article highlights the crucial role of ICE to identify the anatomy associated with different types of cardiac arrhythmias and guide the procedural approach. We wish to thank all the authors for their outstanding contributions.

Pasquale Santangeli, MD, PhD
Electrophysiology Section
Cardiovascular Division
Hospital of the University of Pennsylvania
3400 Spruce Street, 9 Founders Building
Philadelphia, PA 1014, USA

Fermin C. Garcia, MD
Electrophysiology Section
Cardiovascular Division
Hospital of the University of Pennsylvania
3400 Spruce Street, 9 Founders Building
Philadelphia, PA 1014, USA

Luis C. Sáenz, MD
Cardiac Electrophysiology
Fundacion CardioInfantil
Calle 163A # 13B-60
Bogota, Colombia

E-mail addresses:
pasquale.santangeli@gmail.com (P. Santangeli)
Fermin.Garcia@uphs.upenn.edu (F.C. Garcia)
lcsaenz@cardioinfantil.org (L.C. Sáenz)

Card Electrophysiol Clin 13 (2021) xv
https://doi.org/10.1016/j.ccep.2021.04.002
1877-9182/21/© 2021 Published by Elsevier Inc.

How to Use Intracardiac Echocardiography to Recognize Normal Cardiac Anatomy

Houman Khakpour, MD*, Shumpei Mori, MD, PhD, Jason S. Bradfield, MD, Kalyanam Shivkumar, MD, PhD

KEYWORDS

• Cardiac anatomy • Cardiac imaging • Catheter ablation • Intracardiac echocardiography

KEY POINTS

- Intracardiac echocardiography (ICE) provides high-resolution, real-time, near-field imaging of cardiac structures, especially those that are not visualized by fluoroscopy, including intracavitary structures.
- A comprehensive knowledge of 3D cardiac structural anatomy and its attitudinal relationship is fundamental in navigating ICE.
- Standard ICE views and protocols facilitate recognition of normal cardiac anatomy and its variants.

INTRODUCTION

Detailed knowledge of cardiac anatomy is paramount to the success of interventional electrophysiologists, yet it remains underemphasized during electrophysiology training. The advent of highly steerable intracardiac echocardiography (ICE) catheters capable of real-time monitoring and 3-dimensional (3D) electroanatomic map superimposition, along with a heightened focus on radiation-reducing techniques, and visualization limitations of fluoroscopy, has led to increased popularity and utilization of ICE. This article reviews cardiac anatomy as it pertains to commonly used ICE segments and views.

HISTORY AND BACKGROUND OF INTRACARDIAC ECHOCARDIOGRAPHY

Imaging of heart structures with catheter-based tools was explored as early as 1956.[1] Early on, single-crystal probes that were rotating were used to perform cardiac imaging.[2,3] Single-crystal rotating probes were followed by a mechanically rotating 4-element probe developed in the mid-1960s, and a 32-element phased array coil developed in 1969.[4] High-frequency rotating catheter probes in the range of 20 to 30 MHz were subsequently developed for intracoronary assessments.[5] In the 1990s, lower-frequency prototypes (10–12.5 MHz) of these rotating single-element devices were used for the earliest intracardiac investigations.[6] Current commonly used ICE probes are 64-element phased-array 4-way steerable catheters with a frequency range of 5.5 to 10 MHz. Within a cardiac chamber, the probe can be advanced or pulled back, rotated clockwise or counterclockwise, tilted right or left, and flexed anteriorly or posteriorly. Parameters, such as frequency, depth (up to 15 cm), gain, dynamic range, and mechanical index, can be adjusted to optimize the image. The probe produces the classic wedge-shaped image. Images

UCLA Cardiac Arrhythmia Center, David Geffen School of Medicine at UCLA, Los Angeles, CA, USA
* Corresponding author. UCLA Cardiac Arrhythmia Center, 100 Medical Plaza, Suite 660, Los Angeles, CA.
E-mail address: HKhakpour@mednet.ucla.edu

Card Electrophysiol Clin 13 (2021) 273–283
https://doi.org/10.1016/j.ccep.2021.02.001

are displayed as 90° sectors originating from the cardiac chamber where the transducer is located and are commonly displayed with the tip of the catheter to the right of the image and the shaft of the catheter to the left.

IMAGING PROTOCOLS AND STANDARD ECHOCARDIOGRAPHIC VIEWS

Cardiac imaging can be successfully obtained and interpreted with the ICE probe placed in any cardiac chamber, and other adjacent cavities, including vessels and intrapericardial space. However, similar to other echocardiographic modalities, ICE image sectors are not necessarily "attitudinally bound." For example, superior structures of the heart are rarely displayed superiorly on the monitor. In addition, even if ICE displays a similar sectional plane to that obtained from transthoracic echocardiography, the image is visualized with significant rotation. These limitations, along

with its relatively narrow field of view, can prevent operators from appreciating correct anatomic orientation, and in the absence of well-defined standard ICE views, may lead to confusion.

Use of standard echocardiographic views and an in-depth understanding of 3D cardiac anatomy enables the operator to navigate cardiac anatomy with more confidence, monitor for complications and collateral damage in real time, and reduce radiation exposure and procedure duration.[7–9]

In later discussion, the authors review echocardiographic views obtained with the ICE catheter positioned in the mid right atrium (RA) and in the right ventricle (RV) in a para-Hisian region (**Fig. 1**).

INTRACARDIAC ECHOCARDIOGRAPHY POSITION IN THE RIGHT ATRIUM

The initial view obtained with the transducer in the neutral position and the ICE catheter positioned in the mid RA is also referred to as the home view. In

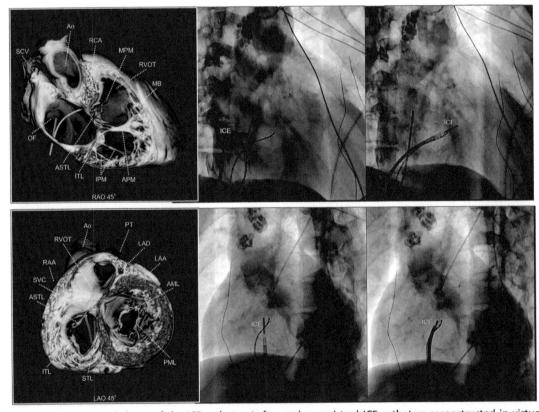

Fig. 1. 3D location and shape of the ICE catheter. Left panels are virtual ICE catheters reconstructed in virtual dissection using computed tomographic data sets. Middle and right panels are fluoroscopic images showing location of the ICE catheter placed in the mid RA and para-Hisian region, respectively. Upper and lower panels are viewed from 45° right anterior oblique (RAO) and left anterior oblique (LAO) directions, respectively. Ao, ascending aorta; APM, anterior papillary muscle; ASTL, anterosuperior tricuspid leaflet; IPM, inferior papillary muscle; ITL, inferior tricuspid leaflet; MB, moderator band; MPM, medial papillary muscle; OF, oval fossa; PML, posterior mitral leaflet; PT, pulmonary trunk; SCV, superior caval vein; STL, septal tricuspid leaflet; SVC, supraventricular crest.

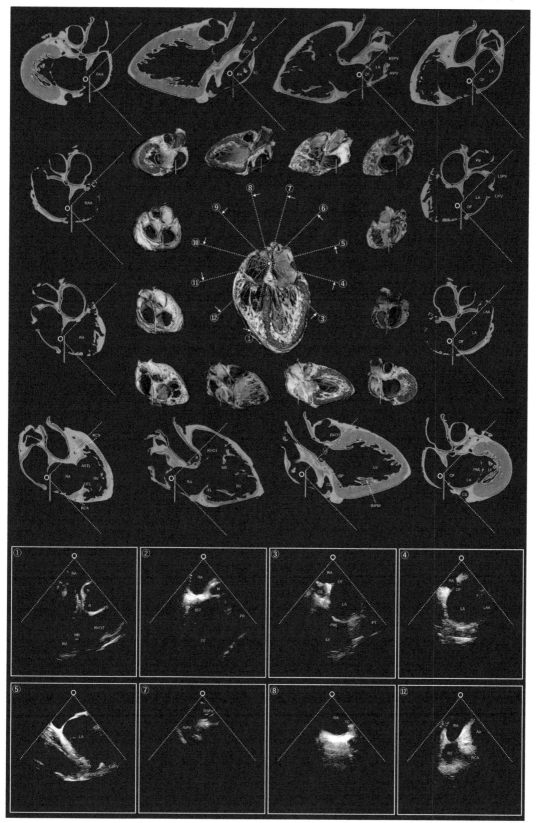

Fig. 2. Rotational demonstration of the representative sections obtained from the ICE catheter placed in the mid RA. Central image is the exact perpendicular section to the ICE catheter. Blue dot represents the axis of the ICE shaft directing toward observer. Along this axis, 12 sets of rotational sections are reconstructed using virtual

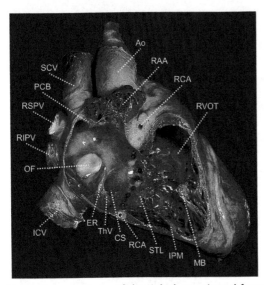

Fig. 3. Gross anatomy of the right heart viewed from the right anterior oblique direction. ER, Eustachian ridge; ICV, inferior caval vein; PCB, precaval bundle; RSPV, right superior pulmonary vein; ThV, Thebesian valve. (Illustration courtesy of UCLA Cardiac Arrhythmia Center, Wallace A. McAlpine MD collection.)

this view, segments of RA, tricuspid valve, and RV are visualized. An oblique view of the aortic valve and proximal ascending aorta can be seen, sometimes needing a slight clockwise rotation (**Fig. 2**, ①, ②). The segments in later discussion review a 360° rotation in a clockwise direction from the mid right atrial position (see **Fig. 2**, ①-②).

Home View: Anatomic Correlation in the Right Atrium

In the RA, the junction between the smooth-walled sinus venarum posteriorly and the pectinated anterior portion is marked by the interior projection of a well-formed muscle bundle, the terminal crest (also known as crista terminalis). The terminal crest is most prominent superiorly and continues in front of the orifice of the superior vena cava (SVC) as a prominent ridge (called arcuate ridge or precaval bundle). The inferior margin of terminal crest continues anterior to the IVC and is reinforced during fetal development by a sheetlike

structure that separates IVC from the atrial appendage. This crescentic structure becomes the Eustachian valve (or ridge), which attaches to the inferior right atrial wall and projects superiorly from the anterior margin of the IVC orifice and is often confluent with valve of the coronary sinus (CS) called the Thebesian valve (**Fig. 3**). Anterior and inferior to this orifice, the trabeculated RA may have considerable pouches, called the sub-Eustachian and sub-Thebesian sinuses. The inferior RA wall, which includes the so-called cavotricuspid isthmus (CTI), extends posteriorly to the orifice of IVC and medially to the ostium of left ventricle (LV) and the CS.

Subtle manipulation of the home view will provide information about the CTI, including its length, presence of pouches (sub-Eustachian sinuses), the prominence of the Eustachian ridge, and the thickness of pectinate muscles, which form the pectinated portion of the inferior RA wall. ICE can be useful in delineating anatomic variations in this region, guide in catheter manipulation during ablation of CTI-dependent atrial flutter, and reduce radiation exposure and ablation time.[10–12]

Home View Clocked: Septal Tricuspid Leaflet and Bundle of His

The attachment of the septal leaflet of the tricuspid valve to the membranous septum demarcates the atrioventricular (RA connection to LV) and interventricular (LV connection to RV) portions of the membranous septum. The membranous septum and the right fibrous trigone together comprise the central fibrous body and are fundamental anatomic landmarks in studying the cardiac conduction system: The AV node is anterosuperior to the CS orifice and is commonly located on the central fibrous body, just posterior to the right fibrous trigone. The penetrating (first) portion of His bundle traverses the atrioventricular portion of the membranous septum, and the branching portion of the His bundle runs in relation to the inferior margin of the membranous septum.

From the home view, clockwise rotation of the ICE catheter allows for excellent visualization of this region. In this view (see **Fig. 2**, ①), RA, tricuspid annulus with septal and inferior leaflets

dissection (color) and virtual ICE (gray scale) images per each 30° rotation. Blue lines indicate virtual ICE catheters. Each section is an image slice viewed from the en-face direction, indicated by arrows, to simulate ICE images. Circles denote the location of the probe, and dotted lines mark the 90° sectors. ICE catheter is nearly parallel to body axis. When rotational scan is started from the home view (), the focus of interest follows the anatomic alignments shown in the central image, including the RV (①, ②), LV (②-③), left atrium (④-⑦), and RA (⑧-⑪). Inferior panels are representative *real* ICE images. Numbers correspond to those in superior *virtual* panels. IMPM, inferomedial papillary muscle; ISP, inferoseptal process; LA, left atrium; MB, moderator band; N, noncoronary aortic sinus; PR, pulmonary root; R, right coronary aortic sinus; RSPV, right superior pulmonary vein; TC, terminal crest.

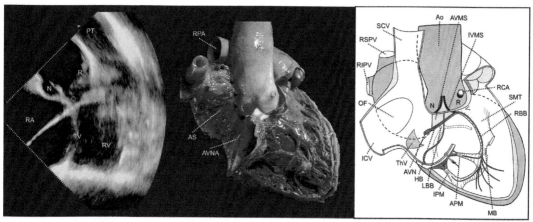

Fig. 4. Home view rotated 90° counterclockwise and corresponding gross anatomy. When home view is rotated 90° counterclockwise (*left panel*), it becomes "attitudinally correct" and facilitates understanding the anatomy. Middle and right panels are representative cardiac illustrations. A His-bundle catheter is placed in this case. Note the RA is removed in the middle panel. AS, atrial septum; AVMS, atrioventricular portion of the membranous septum; AVN, atrioventricular node; AVNA, atrioventricular nodal artery; HB, bundle of His; IVMS, interventricular portion of the membranous septum; LBB, left bundle branch; R, right coronary aortic sinus; RBB, right bundle branch; SMT, septomarginal trabeculation; TV, tricuspid valve. (Illustrations courtesy of UCLA Cardiac Arrhythmia Center, Wallace A. McAlpine MD collection.)

of the tricuspid valve, and a long-axis view of the aorta and the aortic valve are displayed. The noncoronary cusp of the aortic valve (NCC), more suitably called noncoronary aortic sinus from an anatomic perspective, is adjacent to the tricuspid valve septal leaflet, and the right coronary cusp (the right coronary aortic sinus) is anterior to that. In addition, the right ventricular outflow tract (RVOT) in long axis, and the pulmonic valve can also be appreciated in this view. Indeed, a 90° counterclockwise rotation of this ICE image will render it "attitudinally correct" (**Fig. 4**). This view would be of significant value, for example, in catheter ablation of para-Hisian foci. Mapping of the RV basal anteroseptal region for ventricular arrhythmias of para-Hisian origin, corresponding the inferior margin of the membranous septum, can be achieved with ICE guidance, by placing a

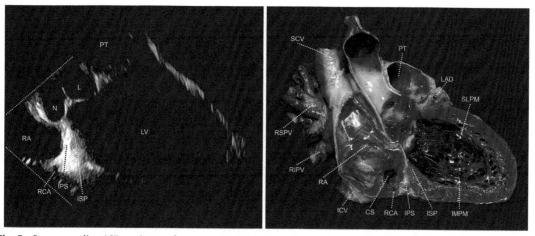

Fig. 5. Corresponding ICE section and gross anatomy. 90° counterclockwise rotation of ICE image (*left panel*) renders it attitudinally correct and facilitates understanding of anatomy. Right panel is a representative cardiac illustration. Relationship between the RA, CS, inferior pyramidal space, inferoseptal process, and LV can be easily appreciated. ICV, inferior caval vein; IPS, inferior pyramidal space; L, left coronary aortic sinus; N, noncoronary aortic sinus; SLPM, superolateral papillary muscle. (Illustration courtesy of UCLA Cardiac Arrhythmia Center, Wallace A. McAlpine MD collection.)

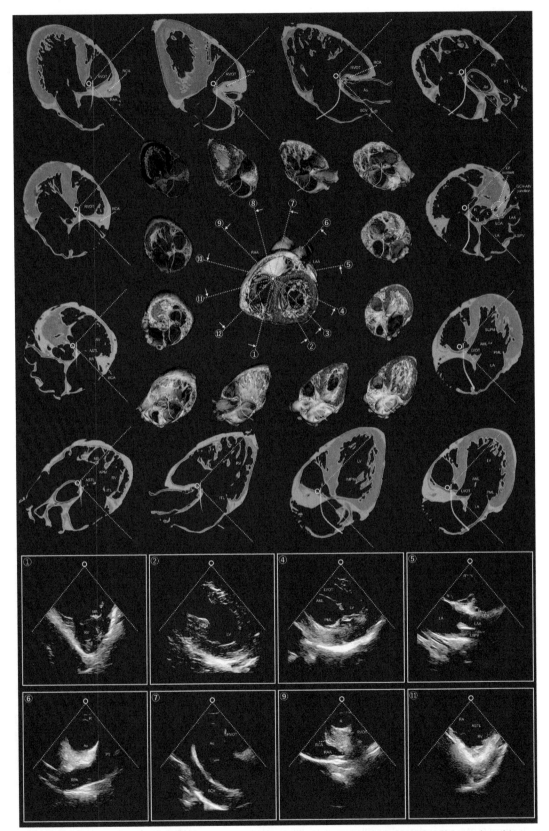

Fig. 6. Rotational demonstration of the representative sections obtained from the ICE catheter placed in para-Hisian region. Central image is the exact perpendicular section to the ICE catheter. Blue dot represents the axis of the ICE shaft directing toward observer. Along this axis, 12 sets of rotational sections are reconstructed

long sheath in the RV and curving the ablation catheter to place it under the septal tricuspid valve leaflet (with either a primary curve or a "reverse S curve" approach).[13]

Further Clockwise Rotation from the Home View

With further clockwise rotation of the ICE catheter positioned in the mid RA, the CS ostium along with the LV outflow tract in the long axis is identified. The NCC is adjacent to the RA and the atrioventricular portion of the membranous septum, and the left coronary cusp (LCC) of the aortic valve (more appropriately called left coronary aortic sinus) can be seen superiorly and leftward to the NCC. Inferior to the NCC, the most inferior and posterior portion of basal LV, the inferoseptal process (also known as the nonattitudinally bound terminology of "posterior superior process"), of LV may be appreciated (see **Fig. 2**, ②). The inferoseptal process is anatomically adjacent to the inferomedial aspect of the RA; the inferior wall of the RA lies above and lateral to the inferoseptal process, which is adjacent to the inferior pyramidal space. The CS orifice is medial to this area (**Fig. 5**). The atrioventricular node artery ascends onto the inferoseptal process crossing within the fat of the pyramidal space. Successful ablation of ventricular arrhythmias arising from this region, with the ablation catheter in the RA or LV guided by ICE, has been performed.[14]

Additional clockwise rotation allows visualization of interatrial septum, CS body, posterior mitral leaflet, and the left atrial appendage (LAA) anteriorly and leftward (see **Fig. 2**, ③-④). Minor adjustments in the catheter tilt can optimize visualization of the oval fossa (fossa ovalis), and the superior and inferior interatrial grooves. Continued clockwise rotation provides more posterior viewing of the left atrium and identifies the left superior (LSPV) and left inferior (LIPV) pulmonary veins in their long axis (see **Fig. 2**, ⑤). LSPV appears superiorly in the image before or on time with LIPV, which is seen inferiorly. As the clockwise movement continues, it will bring into view the posterior/inferior wall of the LA, the descending aorta, and the esophagus (see **Fig. 2**, ⑥). Slight cranial advancement of the probe with continued clockwise torque past the esophageal view will put in view the right inferior pulmonary vein (RIPV) at around the 6 to 7 o'clock display. From the left atrium/RIPV view, a slight clockwise rotation of the catheter will allow visualization of both the inferior and the superior pulmonary veins in a short axis (see **Fig. 2**, ⑦). In this view, the transverse sinus and a short axis of right pulmonary artery (RPA) are also displayed. Advancement of the probe, usually with a slight posterior tilt and right or left tilting, as clockwise rotation is continued, will display the right superior pulmonary vein more longitudinally. Both inferior pulmonary veins are more posterior and inferior to their superior counterparts. Color Doppler can be used to assist with identifying the pulmonary venous inflow.

As clockwise rotation continues, the posterior RA comes into view, and a posterior catheter tilt may optimize SVC and arcuate ridge (precaval bundle) visualization (see **Fig. 2**, ⑧). As the movement continues and the probe scans the lateral and anterior RA wall, the terminal crest is seen as a ridgelike structure, and eventually the right atrial appendage (RAA) is displayed (see **Fig. 2**, ⑨-⑩). With further clockwise rotation, tricuspid valve leaflets and RV will be viewed; right coronary artery (RCA) may also be identified during the rotation. Finally, the home view is once again in display with further rotation.

INTRACARDIAC ECHOCARDIOGRAPHY POSITION THE RIGHT VENTRICULAR LOCATION

From the home view position in the RA, the ICE catheter is anteriorly tilted and then advanced through the tricuspid valve into the RV under fluoroscopy or ICE guidance. When the catheter is in the RV, the anterior steer is released. The position of the ICE catheter at this point approximates a para-Hisian location where the *His* signal is recorded (see **Fig. 1**). This position, referred to in this text as the RV para-Hisian position, provides viewing of the RV inferior wall and infundibulum,

---

using virtual dissection (color) and virtual ICE (gray scale) images. Blue lines indicate virtual ICE catheters. Each section is an image slice viewed from the en-face direction indicated by arrows, to simulate ICE images. Yellow circles denote the location of the probe, and dotted lines mark the 90° sectors. When rotational scan is started from the right ventricular long-axis view (), the focus of interest follows the anatomic alignments shown in the central image, including the RV (①, ②), LV (②-④), aortic root and LAA (⑤), pulmonary trunk (⑥), ascending aorta (⑦), and anterosuperior part of the right atrioventricular groove (⑧-⑪). Inferior panels are representative *real* ICE images. Numbers correspond to those in the superior *virtual* panels. AIV, anterior interventricular vein; GCV, great cardiac vein; LCA, left coronary artery; PV, pulmonary valve, RAVG, right atrioventricular groove; TS, transverse sinus.

and further clockwise rotations move the image sector into the LV, left atrium, short axis of the aortic valve, aorta, pulmonary artery, and pulmonic valve, and back in the RV. In this position, anterior and cranial advancement of the catheter optimizes viewing of the apical structures, and retracting the probe toward the tricuspid valve annulus better characterizes the basal structures. The following sections provide an anatomic correlation, as the ICE catheter is rotated clockwise 360° in the RV para-Hisian position (**Fig. 6**, ①-⑫).

Right Ventricle Papillary Muscles and the Moderator Band

The muscles of the RV may be divided into 3 groups: (1) the papillary muscles of the tricuspid valve, (2) the infundibular muscles, and (3) the trabeculae. The papillary muscles of the tricuspid valve are termed medial (septal), anterior, and inferior. The anterior and inferior papillary muscles, attached to the anterior and inferior walls, respectively, provide insertion for the chordae from nonseptal leaflets of the tricuspid valve. Chordae from the tricuspid valve septal and anterosuperior leaflets are attached with or without the intermediation of small medial papillary muscle to the septal wall. The postero(septal) wall of the RV infundibulum extends from the pulmonic valve attachment inferiorly to the septomarginal trabeculation, which continues to become the moderator band, projecting anteriorly to the site of attachment of the

anterior papillary muscle to the RV anterior wall (see **Figs. 3** and **4**). The right bundle runs within the septomarginal trabeculation to the moderator band, reaching the anterior papillary muscle, where it terminates in the Purkinje system. The moderator band is a source of Purkinje-related ventricular arrhythmias.[15,16] With the ICE catheter in the RV para-Hisian position, RV inferior wall, papillary muscles, and moderator band may be characterized with slight tilt adjustments (see **Fig. 6**, ①).

Left Ventricle Papillary Muscles

Both superolateral and inferomedial papillary muscles (also called by the nonattitudinal terms of anterolateral and posteromedial papillary muscles, respectively) of the LV insert into the intermediate third of the LV; generally, inferomedial papillary muscle originates from inferior to inferolateral wall of the LV, and the superolateral papillary muscle originates from the anterolateral wall (**Fig. 7**). In about two-thirds of hearts, the superolateral papillary muscle is a single structure, and the inferomedial papillary muscle consists of separately based bundles. The superolateral papillary muscle is usually larger, simpler in design, and less tethered to the ventricular wall. The superior and inferior fascicles of the left bundle branch are directed toward superolateral and inferomedial papillary muscles. Both LV papillary muscles are well-described

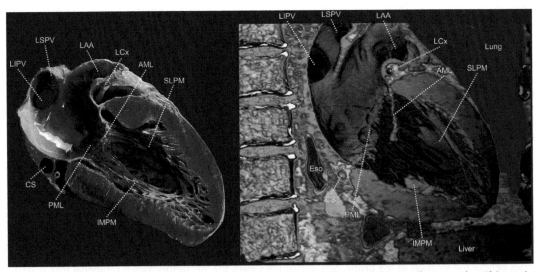

Fig. 7. Representative gross and virtual dissection image showing left ventricular papillary muscles. This section corresponds to echocardiographic 2-chamber view. Note the papillary muscles are aligned in superoinferior fashion (see **Fig. 2**, section ②). Both papillary muscles belong exclusively to the left ventricular free wall, not to the septum. Eso, esophagus; LCx, left circumflex artery. (Illustration courtesy of UCLA Cardiac Arrhythmia Center, Wallace A. McAlpine MD collection.)

sources of non-Purkinje and Purkinje-related ventricular arrhythmias.[17–19]

Gentle clockwise rotation from the above (RV) view will first display the interventricular septum and the LV apex followed by long-axis view of the LV anterior and inferior walls in display (see **Fig. 6**, ②-③). Here, the LV inferomedial papillary muscle can be appreciated in the long axis. Further clockwise torque will display in an oblique view the superolateral papillary muscle, along with the lateral and inferior LV walls, and parts of anterior and posterior leaflets of the mitral valve (see **Fig. 6**, ④).

Left Ventricle Base, Aortic and Pulmonic Valves and Trunk and the Coronary Arteries

Continued clockwise rotation from the above position (superolateral papillary muscle view) puts in display basal portions of the LV and fibrous skeleton of the heart: as torque is applied, the anterior mitral leaflet (AML), lateral followed by medial aspect of the aortomitral continuity (AMC), left ventricular outflow tract (LVOT), LV summit, aortic valve leaflets, and the ostium of the left main coronary artery are visualized (see **Fig. 6**, ④-⑥). Posteriorly, the left atrium and the aorta are displayed during this clockwise rotation.

Short-axis view of the aortic valve is conveniently achieved during the rotation from the superolateral papillary muscle/AML view (see **Fig. 6**, ⑥). The leaflet closest to the probe belongs to RCC with NCC adjacent to that and anterior to the left atrium. LCC is seen leftward on this view and is anterior to the LAA. The left main coronary artery and its ostium can be appreciated from this view. A left anterior descending artery (LAD) course as it runs in the interventricular groove can be followed by counterclockwise movements of the probe. Pulmonic trunk running between the aortic root and the LAA may be characterized as well (see **Fig. 6**, ⑥-⑦). Two leaflets of the pulmonic valve, the left (immediately adjacent to the LCC) and nonadjacent (anterior) pulmonic leaflets, are in view with minor adjustments to this position. Posterior to the aortic sinuses, the left pulmonary veins may be identified (see **Fig. 6**, ⑥). As clockwise rotation continues, cranial advancement of the probe in the RVOT displays a long-axis view of the ascending aorta. RCC and NCC of the aortic valve may be identified. Posteriorly, segments of LA, RSPV, and RPA are appreciated (see **Fig. 6**, ⑦). Further clockwise torque displays ostium and proximal course of the RCA and long-axis views of the ascending aorta and SVC followed by RAA (see **Fig. 6**, ⑧-⑩). Finally, tricuspid valve leaflets followed by papillary muscles and moderator band will be in view again as the probe completes its 360° rotation (see **Fig. 6**, ⑪-⑫).

OTHER USEFUL VIEWS
Probe in the Right Atrial Appendage

With the probe in the superior RAA, slight anterior tilt may allow visualization of the RCA ostium and its proximal portion.[20] Clockwise rotation allows visualization of the aortic valve (oblique/long axis) with NCC and LCC in view and anteriorly of the pulmonic valve in short axis (**Fig. 8**). Identification of aortic and pulmonic valve leaflets using ICE (placed in the RAA or the RV position) can be

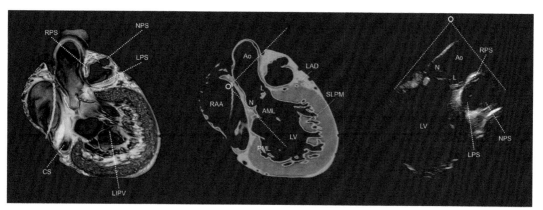

Fig. 8. Representative sections from the medial RAA. Virtual dissection (*left panel*), virtual ICE (*middle panel*) with virtual ICE catheter (*blue*), and real ICE images (*right panel*). Transverse image of the pulmonary root with longitudinal section of the ascending aorta is demonstrated. Circles denote the location of the probe, and dotted lines mark the 90° sectors. LPS, left adjacent pulmonary sinus; NPS, nonadjacent pulmonary sinus; RPS, right adjacent pulmonary sinus.

advantageous during catheter ablation of outflow tract ventricular arrhythmias.[21]

Probe in the Main Pulmonary Artery

From the RVOT, the probe can be carefully advanced into the pulmonary artery. With an anterior tilt, the LAA can be visualized with clarity. Clockwise and counterclockwise rotation of the probe allows for visualization of the proximal and distal parts of the LAA, respectively.

Probe in the Pericardial Space

Percutaneous intrapericardial cardiac echo (PICE) has been performed in patients undergoing epicardial catheter ablation. PICE images provide views of the heart from the pericardial sinuses. This approach provides high-resolution imaging of structures that may not be easily seen with conventional ICE probe positions.[22]

SUMMARY

ICE provides high-quality, real-time near-field images of cardiac structures. Knowledge of cardiac anatomy and its attitudinal relationship is fundamental in navigating ICE images. Familiarity with standard views from the RA and RV vantage points facilitates recognition of cardiac anatomy and provides guidance in electrophysiology procedures.

DISCLOSURE

None.

REFERENCES

1. Cieszynski T. Intracardiac method for the investigation of structure of the heart with the aid of ultrasonics. Arch Immunol Ther Exp (Warsz) 1960;8: 551–7. Available at: https://pubmed.ncbi.nlm.nih.gov/13693633/. Accessed November 6, 2020.
2. Kossoff G. Diagnostic applications of ultrasound in cardiology. Australas Radiol 1966;10(2):101–6.
3. Kimoto S, Omoto R, Tsunemoto M, et al. Ultrasonic tomography of the liver and detection of heart atrial septal defect with the aid of ultrasonic intravenous probes. Ultrasonics 1964;2(2):82–6.
4. Bom N, Lancée CT, van Egmond FC. An ultrasonic intracardiac scanner. Ultrasonics 1972;10(2):72–6.
5. Pandian NG, Kreis A, Brockway B, et al. Ultrasound angioscopy: real-time, two-dimensional, intraluminal ultrasound imaging of blood vessels. Am J Cardiol 1988;62(7):493–4.
6. Pandian NG, Kreis A, Weintraub A, et al. Real-time intravascular ultrasound imaging in humans. Am J Cardiol 1990;65(20):1392–6.
7. Marrouche NF, Martin DO, Wazni O, et al. Phased-array intracardiac echocardiography monitoring during pulmonary vein isolation in patients with atrial fibrillation: impact on outcome and complications. Circulation 2003;107(21):2710–6.
8. Ren JF, Marchlinski FE. Monitoring and early diagnosis of procedural complications. In: Ren JF, Marchlinski FE, Callans DJ, et al, editors. Practical intracardiac echocardiography in electrophysiology. Wiley-Blackwell; 2008. p. 180–207.
9. Razminia M, Willoughby MC, Demo H, et al. Fluoroless catheter ablation of cardiac arrhythmias: a 5-year experience. Pacing Clin Electrophysiol 2017; 40(4):425–33.
10. Morton JB, Sanders P, Davidson NC, et al. Phased-array intracardiac echocardiography for defining cavotricuspid isthmus anatomy during radiofrequency ablation of typical atrial flutter. J Cardiovasc Electrophysiol 2003;14(6):591–7.
11. BENCSIK G, PAP R, MAKAI A, et al. Randomized trial of intracardiac echocardiography during cavotricuspid isthmus ablation. J Cardiovasc Electrophysiol 2012;23(9):996–1000.
12. Hisazaki K, Kaseno K, Miyazaki S, et al. Intra-procedural evaluation of the cavo-tricuspid isthmus anatomy with different techniques: comparison of angiography and intracardiac echocardiography. Heart Vessels 2019;34(10):1703–9.
13. Enriquez A, Tapias C, Rodriguez D, et al. How to map and ablate parahisian ventricular arrhythmias. Heart Rhythm 2018;15(8):1268–74.
14. Santangeli P, Hutchinson MD, Supple GE, et al. Right atrial approach for ablation of ventricular arrhythmias arising from the left posterior-superior process of the left ventricle. Circ Arrhythmia Electrophysiol 2016; 9(7). https://doi.org/10.1161/CIRCEP.116.004048.
15. Sadek MM, Benhayon D, Sureddi R, et al. Idiopathic ventricular arrhythmias originating from the moderator band: electrocardiographic characteristics and treatment by catheter ablation. Heart Rhythm 2015;12(1):67–75.
16. Anter E, Buxton AE, Silverstein JR, et al. Idiopathic ventricular fibrillation originating from the moderator band. J Cardiovasc Electrophysiol 2013;24(1):97–100.
17. Doppalapudi H, Yamada T, McElderry HT, et al. Ventricular tachycardia originating from the posterior papillary muscle in the left ventricle: a distinct clinical syndrome. Circ Arrhythmia Electrophysiol 2008;1(1):23–9.
18. Yamada T, McElderry HT, Okada T, et al. Idiopathic focal ventricular arrhythmias originating from the anterior papillary muscle in the left ventricle. J Cardiovasc Electrophysiol 2009; 20(8):866–72.
19. Akihiko N. Purkinje-related arrhythmias part I: monomorphic ventricular tachycardias. Pacing Clin Electrophysiol 2011;34(5):624–50.

20. Enriquez A, Saenz LC, Rosso R, et al. Use of intracardiac echocardiography in interventional cardiology working with the anatomy rather than fighting it. Circulation 2018;137(21):2278–94.

21. Ehdaie A, Liu F, Cingolani E, et al. How to use intracardiac echocardiography to guide catheter ablation of outflow tract ventricular arrhythmias. Heart Rhythm 2020;17(8):1405–10.

22. Horowitz BN, Vaseghi M, Mahajan A, et al. Percutaneous intrapericardial echocardiography during catheter ablation: a feasibility study. Heart Rhythm 2006;3(11):1275–82.

Intracardiac Echocardiography to Guide Catheter Ablation of Ventricular Arrhythmias in Ischemic Cardiomyopathy

Pierre C. Qian, MBBS, PhD[a], Usha B. Tedrow, MD, MS[b],*

KEYWORDS

- Intracardiac echocardiography • Ischemic cardiomyopathy • Ventricular arrhythmias
- Catheter ablation

KEY POINTS

- Intracardiac echocardiography (ICE) is useful for intraprocedural assessment of the extent of ischemic myocardial scar and its relationship to cardiac structures, such as papillary muscles and valves.
- Real-time visualization of the catheter position using ICE is helpful for maneuvering catheters to critical sites for mapping and ablation.
- ICE allows continuous monitoring of ablation lesion creation and early detection of complications.
- Image integration of ICE with other modalities, such as computed tomography/MRI and electroanatomic mapping, provides enhanced understanding of substrate and arrhythmia mechanisms.

 Video content accompanies this article at http://www.cardiacep.theclinics.com.

INTRODUCTION

Ventricular arrhythmias in patients with ischemic cardiomyopathy often arise from reentry circuits involving slow conduction of surviving myocytes in regions of dense fibrosis. Anatomically, these regions can exhibit thinning, akinesis, and, at times, aneurysm formation. Ventricular arrhythmias in ischemic heart disease can also be the result of automaticity in areas of damaged Purkinje fibers or partially fibrosed papillary muscles. An appreciation of anatomy together with electrophysiological characteristics helps identify the arrhythmogenic substrate and mechanism of arrhythmia to guide catheter ablation therapy. Intracardiac echocardiography (ICE) is a useful modality that provides anatomical information which can be integrated with electroanatomical mapping and provides real-time visualization of the ablation catheter and lesion formation. In this review, the authors discuss the applications of ICE for mapping and ablation of ventricular arrhythmias arising from ischemic substrates.

Funding: None.
Conflicts of Interest: Dr U.B. Tedrow has received speaking honoraria from Abbott Medical, Biosense Webster, Medtronic, and Boston Scientific, Inc, as well as consulting fees from Thermedical Inc.
[a] Department of Cardiology, Westmead Hospital, Sydney, Australia; [b] Cardiovascular Division, Department of Medicine, Brigham and Women's Hospital, 75 Francis Street, Boston, MA 02115, USA
* Corresponding author.
E-mail address: utedrow@bwh.harvard.edu

Card Electrophysiol Clin 13 (2021) 285–292
https://doi.org/10.1016/j.ccep.2021.02.002

DEFINING ISCHEMIC MYOCARDIAL SCAR

Postmyocardial infarction scar is often readily seen on ICE as a region of hypokinesis or akinesis and tends to be thinner than the surrounding healthy myocardium. Given the increased reflection of ultrasound by regions of intramyocardial fibrosis, intramyocardial scar can be appreciated as a hyperechoic region.[1] The signal intensity on ICE correlates with regions of scar by voltage criteria identified at electroanatomic mapping in patients.[2] Thinned aneurysmal regions of the ventricle are important to explore, as most circuitry for reentrant ventricular arrhythmias arise from regions of myocardial scar ≤5 mm in thickness.[3] Using ICE (Soundstar; Biosense Webster, Irvine, CA, USA) in conjunction with Cartosound (Biosense Webster), the ventricular endocardium can be delineated to generate a 3-dimensional (3D) volume that is incorporated into the electroanatomic map. Regions of ventricular scar can also be represented in a similar fashion (**Fig. 1**). Intracardiac echocardiography can be useful for directing contact mapping to these high-yield areas.

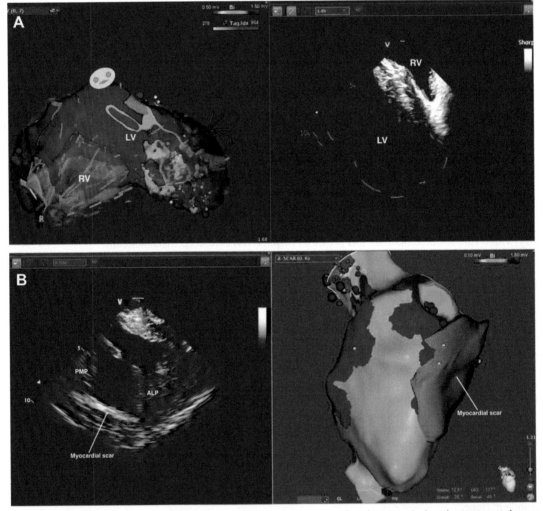

Fig. 1. Inferolateral myocardial infarction scar on ICE. (*A*) A patient with ischemic apical and anteroseptal aneurysm with prior failed endocardial catheter ablation. At redo catheter ablation procedure, ICE demonstrated the extent of the anteroapical aneurysm, the septal extent of which had not been previously appreciated. The Cartosound (Biosense Webster) -generated 3D volumes can be coregistered with segmented cardiac CT to overlay the region of wall thinning (*brown*) onto the electroanatomic map. (*B*) Another patient where a thinned and echogenic ischemic scar is visualized between the posteromedial papillary muscle (PMP) and the anterolateral papillary muscle (ALP). The scar itself can be contoured using Cartosound to be represented as a 3D volume to guide catheter ablation.

UNDERSTANDING REGIONAL ANATOMY AND BARRIERS TO EFFECTIVE RADIOFREQUENCY ABLATION

Knowing the regional anatomy associated with ischemic scars and the barriers that might prevent successful catheter ablation is helpful. Regions of calcification and the presence of overlying chronic laminated thrombus often complicate anteroapical aneurysm and can prevent successful radiofrequency energy delivery into these areas. Intramyocardial calcification can be found in 70% of

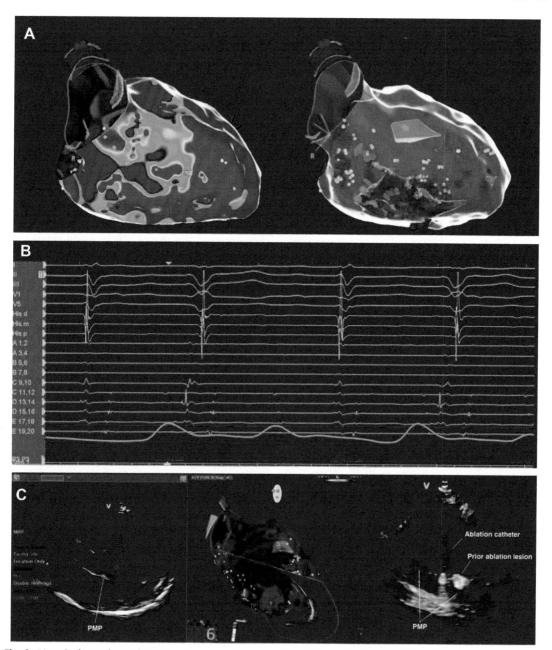

Fig. 2. Ventricular tachycardia arising from papillary muscles within ischemic scar. This patient had extensive anteroseptal dense scar (*A*, *red* ≤0.5 mV) surrounding an akinetic PMP. Interesting, diastolic double potentials were recorded on the PMP using PentaRay (*B*) at the site of the shadowed catheter in (*A*), suggestive for localized reentry, leading to premature ventricular contractions alternating with exit block from the papillary muscle. Using ICE, the ablation catheter was maneuvered to target substrate on the PMP. The ICE sector fan is shown intersecting ablation lesions on the tip of one of the heads of the PMP (first 2 images in *C*). The rightmost image in (*C*) demonstrates an echogenic ablation lesion on the lateral aspect of the lateral head of the PMP, and the ablation catheter moved to an adjacent location between 2 heads of the PMP to deliver another lesion.

patients with ischemic cardiomyopathy and ventricular tachycardia (VT) and corresponds to regions of inexcitability associated with critical substrates for reentrant VT.[4] Both automatic and reentrant circuits can involve the papillary muscles adjacent to or within the ischemic scar. Infarction may involve the papillary muscle itself, which may be akinetic and fibrosed, or relatively spared and adjacent to infarcted myocardium. In addition, the posteromedial papillary muscle may shield critical ischemic substrate, requiring an epicardial approach.[5] Definition of papillary muscle anatomy and their relation to thinned ischemic scar is useful for targeting these arrhythmias (see **Fig. 1**; **Fig. 2**, Video 1). The complexity and bulk of the papillary muscles, which can be readily appreciated on ICE, are predictors of successful ablation for foci or circuits involving these structures.[6]

For basal inferior aneurysms, the extent of the superior-posterior process of the left ventricle and adjacent cardiac crux region can be assessed with ICE. Complete exploration of this region is important, as it can harbor critical arrhythmogenic substrates. Catheter reach may be challenging in this region, and ICE is often helpful to assess catheter-to-tissue contact. A view from the right atrium is often effective for visualizing this region and can help assess whether critical sites are accessible from a right atrial approach[7] (Video 2).

The definition of valve annuli, aortomitral continuity, coronary cusps, and proximal coronary arteries is useful for targeting ventricular arrhythmias originating from periaortic substrates. If ICE is used in conjunction with Cartosound (Biosense Webster), the contours of the outflow tract region, aortic valve annulus, each coronary cusp, and ostium of the left main coronary artery can be integrated into the electroanatomic map to facilitate mapping and ablation. Inferior infarcts often exhibit perimitral circuits that require ablation up to the mitral valve annulus. The plane of the mitral valve is clearly defined on ICE and marked on the electroanatomic mapping system using Cartosound. The annular position of the ablation catheter can be further affirmed on ICE. In the case of inferoposterior aneurysms, the posteromedial papillary muscles may at times block easy access with a mapping catheter into the aneurysmal portion of the ventricle, a situation easily appreciated on ICE mapping of the left ventricle. Anteroseptal aneurysms can extend much further apically and septally than initially suspected (see **Fig. 1**), and ICE can be used to ensure complete aneurysm mapping. ICE can also be used to appreciate unforeseen unusual anatomic situations that may have arisen in a given patient. For example, the use of ICE to guide ablation of VT arising from a left ventricular aneurysm in a patient after surgical repair using the Dor procedure has been reported.[8] Because of partial dehiscence of the endoventricular patch, the catheter was navigated under ICE guidance beneath the patch to the successfully ablate VT (**Fig. 3**).

MULTIMODALITY IMAGE INTEGRATION

By using ICE to construct volumes in 3D space, structures such as cardiac chambers, papillary muscles, valves, and coronary vessel ostia can

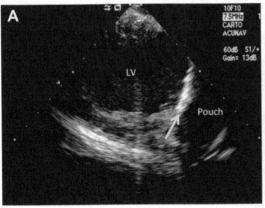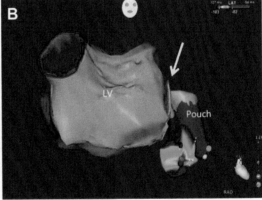

Fig. 3. Catheter ablation of substrate under partially dehisced Dor patch repair of ischemic apical aneurysm. ICE and integration with electroanatomic mapping system using Cartosound (Biosense Webster) enabled delineation and generation of the 3D volume representing the apical aneurysm partially excluded by the dehisced endoventricular patch. Under ICE guidance, the ablation catheter was maneuvered beneath the endoventricular patch to map and successfully ablate the ventricular tachycardia at the earliest activation site (orange dot represents the successful ablation site). (Images are adapted from Tokuda et al. 2014,[8] reproduced with permission from the publisher.)

be rapidly created in a noncontact fashion using Cartosound (Biosense Webster), enabling accurate registrations of the electroanatomic map with cardiac computed tomography (CT) or MRI to integrate myocardial tissue characterization and wall thickness information for delineation of arrhythmogenic substrates. With image processing using third-party segmentation software, such as MUSIC (IHU Liryc, Bordeaux, France) and ADAS 3D (ADAS3D SL Medical, Barcelona, Spain), regions of thinned myocardium and potential VT channels can be identified. The course of the coronary vessels and phrenic nerve can also be defined to guide epicardial ablation (**Fig. 4**).

MONITORING CATHETER STABILITY, LESION FORMATION, AND COMPLICATIONS

The consistency of tissue contact during catheter ablation is essential for lesion creation. In particular, ablation on top of and at the base of the papillary muscles, aneurysmal myocardium, and septal aspects of the left ventricular outflow tract in particular can be challenging. Tactile feedback is confounded by interaction of the catheter shaft with the valvular apparatus, and contact force may be poor or highly variable, especially if the desired ablation site is on the papillary muscle itself. Visualization of the catheter tip and its relation to these intracavitary structures provides an understanding of whether the tip is in good contact and can help navigate the catheter to achieve a stable position in the desired location. Lesion formation may be observable as an expanding hyperechoic region because of microbubble formation within the heated myocardium.[9] Steam pop owing to overheating of tissue above the boiling point is associated with rapid expansion of the hyperechoic region and venting of steam, visualized as a shower of microbubbles into the circulation. These microbubbles may be detectable

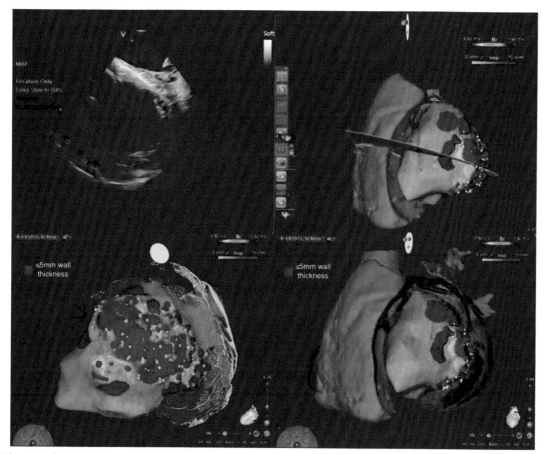

Fig. 4. Multimodality image integration to guide substrate modification. Using ICE, 3D volumes of cardiac chambers, papillary muscles, aortic valve cusps, and coronary ostia can be rapidly acquired without the need for contact mapping (*top left; top right*). This facilitates accurate coregistration of other imaging modalities, such as cardiac CT, which can be segmented, in this case using MUSIC (IHU Liryc), to generate cardiac chambers, regions of wall thinning, coronary arteries, phrenic nerve, device leads, and other structures of interest. In this example, regions of wall thinning (≤5 mm) are overlaid on the electroanatomic map to guide mapping and catheter ablation (*bottom left; bottom right*).

on ICE, but inaudible[10] (**Fig. 5**). Pericardial effusion from cardiac perforation is rapidly detected, allowing for immediate counteractive measures to be undertaken. Occasionally, sheath or catheter-related thrombus is detected on ICE despite intraprocedural anticoagulation. In these instances, withdrawal of the catheter and sheath from the transeptal puncture with concurrent sheath aspiration can usually prevent thromboembolism.[11] In 1 reported case whereby a right atrial thrombus at the transeptal site was detected, ICE-guided direct aspiration of the thrombus was successful.[12]

CLINICAL OUTCOMES

Randomized clinical trial data of using ICE for mapping and ablation of ischemic substrates are not available; however, a propensity matched analysis of retrospective health insurance data suggested a lower rate of repeat VT ablation when ICE is used in patients with ischemic cardiomyopathy (13.06% vs 20.34% over 12 months; $P \leq .01$).[13] Rates of rehospitalization with VT and

procedural complications did not differ significantly whether ICE was used or not in the ischemic cardiomyopathy subgroup in this study. In patients with defibrillators undergoing VT ablation, ICE use was associated with reduced rates of all-cause hospitalization, as well as hospitalization for cardiovascular disease or VT.[14] The use of ICE has enabled reduction or elimination of fluoroscopy use for catheter ablation for a range of arrhythmias, including VT, without negatively impacting procedural efficacy or safety.[15] Prospective studies on the use of ICE for mapping and catheter ablation of ischemic VT are required.

FUTURE DIRECTIONS

New methods for delineating scar by quantifying regional myocardial contraction, such as using speckle tracking or strain echocardiography measures, may improve the detection of substrates for catheter ablation and for assessment of ablation lesion dimensions.[16,17] 3D ICE has shown feasibility and may improve visualization of regional

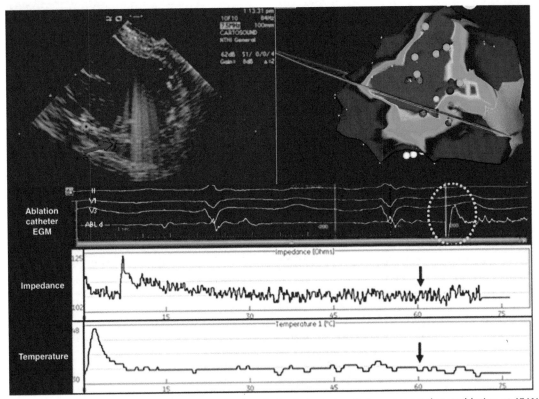

Fig. 5. Detection of silent steam pops. ICE monitoring during irrigated radiofrequency catheter ablation at 45 W. The green circle on the ultrasound image denotes the cross-section of the catheter tip by the ICE sector using Cartosound (Biosense Webster). At 61 seconds of ablation, a jet of microbubbles vents from the ablation lesion (*arrow*) without audible sound. The impedance and temperature tracings were also unremarkable, although the ablation electrode recorded noise that coincided with the event (*circle*). (The images were adapted from Tokuda et al. 2013,[10] reproduced with permission from the publisher.)

anatomy to guide catheter ablation.[18] Prospective studies using ICE for ventricular scar delineation and guidance of catheter ablation are needed to demonstrate the impact of this imaging modality on procedural outcomes.

SUMMARY

ICE provides a real-time means to examine cardiac anatomy, detect myocardial scar and wall thinning, identify barriers to successful radiofrequency ablation, ensure catheter stability, monitor thermal lesion formation, and assist with early detection of complications, thereby arming the proceduralist with more information to tackle ventricular arrhythmias in patients with ischemic cardiomyopathy. The use of ICE for catheter ablation of ventricular arrhythmias has been associated with improved clinical efficacy outcomes in retrospective studies. Prospective studies are required to establish the value and cost-effectiveness of routine use of this technology.

CLINICS CARE POINTS

- Appreciation of the location of scar substrate and regional cardiac anatomy is important in guiding catheter ablation of VT in ischemic cardiomyopathy.

- Intracardiac echography (ICE) can provide real-time assessment of cardiac anatomy and myocardial scar, and identify barriers to successful radiofrequency ablation.

- The use of ICE permits assessment of catheter stability which is particularly challenging on intracavitary structures, monitors thermal lesion formation, detects bleeding and thrombotic complications, and potentially reduces or eliminates fluoroscopy use.

- Familiarity of proceduralists with ICE will enable access to an important tool that provides additional information to facilitate the diagnosis and catheter ablation treatment of ventricular arrhythmias in patients with ischemic cardiomyopathy.

SUPPLEMENTARY DATA

Supplementary data related to this article can be found online at https://doi.org/10.1016/j.ccep.2021.02.002.

REFERENCES

1. Picano E, Pelosi G, Marzilli M, et al. In vivo quantitative ultrasonic evaluation of myocardial fibrosis in humans. Circulation 1990;81:58–64.
2. Hussein A, Jimenez A, Ahmad G, et al. Assessment of ventricular tachycardia scar substrate by intracardiac echocardiography. Pacing Clin Electrophysiol 2014;37:412–21.
3. Komatsu Y, Jadidi A, Sacher F, et al. Relationship between MDCT-imaged myocardial fat and ventricular tachycardia substrate in arrhythmogenic right ventricular cardiomyopathy. J Am Heart Assoc 2014;3:e000935.
4. Alyesh Daniel M, Siontis Konstantinos C, Sharaf Dabbagh G, et al. Postinfarction myocardial calcifications on cardiac computed tomography. Circ Arrhythm Electrophysiol 2019;12:e007023.
5. Enriquez A, Briceno D, Tapias C, et al. Ischemic ventricular tachycardia from below the posteromedial papillary muscle, a particular entity: substrate characterization and challenges for catheter ablation. Heart Rhythm 2019;16:1174–81.
6. Yokokawa M, Good E, Desjardins B, et al. Predictors of successful catheter ablation of ventricular arrhythmias arising from the papillary muscles. Heart rhythm 2010;7:1654–9.
7. Santangeli P, Hutchinson Mathew D, Supple Gregory E, et al. Right atrial approach for ablation of ventricular arrhythmias arising from the left posterior-superior process of the left ventricle. Circ Arrhythm Electrophysiol 2016;9:e004048.
8. Tokuda M, Manlucu J, Brancato S, et al. Catheter ablation of ventricular tachycardia beneath an endoventricular patch. Circulation 2014;130:801–2.
9. Wright M, Harks E, Deladi S, et al. Characteristics of radiofrequency catheter ablation lesion formation in real time in vivo using near field ultrasound imaging. JACC: Clin Electrophysiol 2018;4:1062–72.
10. Tokuda M, Tedrow UB, Stevenson WG. Silent steam pop detected by intracardiac echocardiography. Heart Rhythm 2013;10:1558–9.
11. Blendea D, Barrett CD, Heist EK, et al. Right atrial thrombus aspiration guided by intracardiac echocardiography during catheter ablation for atrial fibrillation. Circ Arrhythm Electrophysiol 2009;2:e18–20.
12. Ren J-F, Marchlinski FE, Callans DJ. Left atrial thrombus associated with ablation for atrial fibrillation: identification with intracardiac echocardiography. J Am Coll Cardiol 2004;43:1861–7.
13. Field ME, Gold MR, Reynolds MR, et al. Real-world outcomes of ventricular tachycardia catheter ablation with versus without intracardiac echocardiography. J Cardiovasc Electrophysiol 2020;31:417–22.

14. Field ME, Goldstein L, Yu Lee SH, et al. Intracardiac echocardiography use and outcomes after catheter ablation of ventricular tachycardia. J Comp Eff Res 2020;9:375–85.
15. Yang L, Sun G, Chen X, et al. Meta-analysis of zero or near-zero fluoroscopy use during ablation of cardiac arrhythmias. Am J Cardiol 2016;118:1511–8.
16. Yue Y, Clark JW Jr, Khoury DS. Speckle tracking in intracardiac echocardiography for the assessment of myocardial deformation. IEEE Trans Biomed Eng 2009;56:416–25.
17. Bunting E, Papadacci C, Wan E, et al. Cardiac lesion mapping in vivo using intracardiac myocardial elastography. IEEE Trans Ultrason Ferroelectr Freq Control 2018;65:14–20.
18. Silvestry FE, Kadakia MB, Willhide J, et al. Initial experience with a novel real-time three-dimensional intracardiac ultrasound system to guide percutaneous cardiac structural interventions: a phase 1 feasibility study of volume intracardiac echocardiography in the assessment of patients with structural heart disease undergoing percutaneous transcatheter therapy. J Am Soc Echocardiogr 2014;27:978–83.

Utility of Intracardiac Echocardiography to Guide Transseptal Catheterization for Different Electrophysiology Procedures

Deep Chandh Raja, MBBS, MD[a], Prashanthan Sanders, MBBS, PhD[b], Rajeev Kumar Pathak, MBBS, PhD[a],*

KEYWORDS

- Intracardiac echocardiography • Transseptal catheterization • Electrophysiology procedures
- Catheter ablation

KEY POINTS

- Transseptal catherization is an important step to access the left atrium and the left ventricle. Use of intracardiac echocardiography (ICE) aids in obtaining a transseptal catherization circumventing the need for transesophageal echocardiography and minimizing the need for fluoroscopy.
- The key advantages of ICE during transseptal access are appreciation of live anatomy of the superior-to-inferior and anterior-to-posterior extent of the interatrial septum and relation to adjacent structures like the aorta, left atrial appendage, left pulmonary veins and the posterior left atrial wall.
- ICE aids in live monitoring of electrophysiological procedures such as catheter ablations, left atrial appendage closures, left ventricular endocardial electrode implantations, and endomyocardial biopsies.

INTRODUCTION

The heart is a 4-dimensional structure, composed of 3 spatial dimensions of shape and one temporal dimension of motion. Many technological advances in the field of imaging, such as cardiac computed tomography (CT), MRI, and electroanatomical mapping have enhanced our ability to visualize, map, and navigate in the heart. Intracardiac echocardiography (ICE) remains an important modality for real-time imaging. Over the last 2 decades, the ability to visualize live cardiac anatomy using ICE while mapping the intracardiac structures has given an edge to the operator in understanding the complex structures such as intracavitary structures such as papillary muscles and the outflow tracts and their attitudinal relationship to adjacent cardiac structures including the coronary vessels.[1] The efficacy and safety of lesions delivered during a radiofrequency ablation can also be monitored with live imaging on ICE.[2]

The utility of ICE has evolved to achieving transseptal catheterization of the left atrium (LA), even without the need for fluoroscopy.[3] LA access is critical for an electrophysiologist for performing ablation in the LA and in some cases for the left ventricle (LV). This article focusses on utilities of ICE for diverse electrophysiology (EP) procedures, such as ablation for atrial fibrillation (AF), left atrial appendage (LAA) closure, access to the mitral annulus for ablation of accessory pathways, and

a Department of Cardiology, Australian National University and Canberra hospital, Canberra, Australian Capital Territory, Australia; b University of Adelaide and Royal Adelaide Hospital, Adelaide, Australia
* Corresponding author. Cardiac Electrophysiology Unit, Department of Cardiology, Canberra Hospital, Yamba Drive, Garran, Australian Capital Territory 2605, Australia.
E-mail address: rajeev.pathak@anu.edu.au

Card Electrophysiol Clin 13 (2021) 293–301
https://doi.org/10.1016/j.ccep.2021.02.003
1877-9182/21/© 2021 Elsevier Inc. All rights reserved.

access to different regions of the LV for various EP procedures.

USE OF INTRACARDIAC ECHOCARDIOGRAPHY IN ATRIAL FIBRILLATION ABLATION

AF is the most common arrhythmia needing medical intervention. Catheter ablation utilizing both thermal and nonthermal energies have shown reasonable reduction in the recurrence rate of AF.[4] Among the various ablation strategies, pulmonary vein isolation (PVI) has become the standard of care for addressing paroxysmal atrial fibrillation[5] (**Figs. 1–3**). For persistent AF the strategies adopted in addition to PVI are posterior wall isolation, elimination of complex fractionated electrograms, addressing the nonpulmonary vein triggers, and modulation of ganglionic plexi.[6] Irrespective of the strategy adopted, each of them requires visualization of the left atrial anatomy for which ICE is incredibly useful.

ICE enables the operator to visualize the LAA in both the short and the long axes. As the morphology of LAA can be appreciated in-depth, the presence of LA and LAA clot can be reliably ruled out before attempting an access into the LA. For transseptal access using ICE, the plane of the pulmonary veins in the atrial septal view is a good position to attempt puncture of interatrial septum (IAS) for purpose of PVI (see **Fig. 1**). A more anterior plane would lead to visualization of the aortic sinuses, and puncture in this plane should be avoided. The live monitoring of the left atrial space between the IAS and the LA posterior wall gives the operator the confidence to maneuver catheters to a safe extent so as not to puncture the LA wall. Lipomatous hypertrophy of the atrial septum, septal aneurysm, persistent left superior vena cava, atrial septal occlusion devices, fibrosed atrial septal secondary to surgeries or redo procedures, atrial myxomas, and atrial septal defects might pose significant challenges where the utility of ICE is all the more important in understanding the exact region of fossa ovalis to obtain access into the LA.[7–10]

In addition, visualization of the LA structures such as pulmonary veins and its relation with LAA is useful for wide antral ablation for PVI. Variations in the anatomy of the pulmonary veins like common Os and supernumerary veins are critical to appreciate while trying to electrically isolate them. ICE gives valuable information such as ensuring contact of the ablation catheter with the

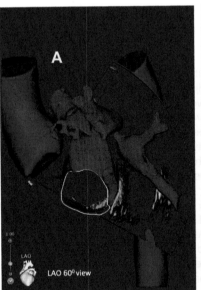
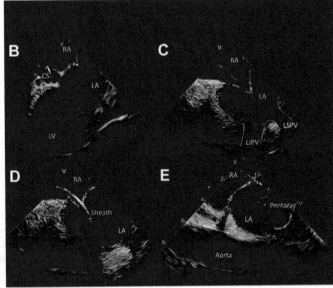

Fig. 1. *The "septal" view and steps in transseptal access for pulmonary vein isolation procedure*: panel A shows the real-time integration of the echocardiographic section (CARTOSOUND) with cardiac CT geometry (CARTO-SEG) while attempting a transseptal access; panel B shows the long-axis view showing the midposition of the transseptal needle across the superoinferior length of the interatrial septum; panel C shows the preferred view to perform the transseptal puncture; panel D shows a deflectable sheath placed across the septum in the LA cavity; panel E shows the hockey-stick shape of the deflectable mapping catheter (Pentaray) in the LA cavity. CS, coronary sinus; LA, left atrium; LAO, left anterior oblique; LIPV, left inferior pulmonary vein; LSPV, left superior pulmonary vein; LV, left ventricle; RA, right atrium.

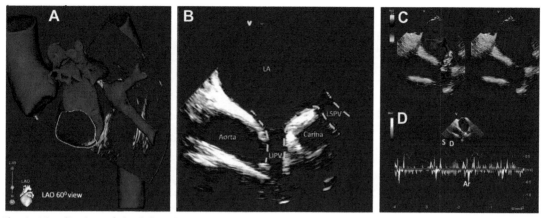

Fig. 2. *Visualization of the left pulmonary veins*: panel A shows the real-time integration of the echocardiographic section (CARTOSOUND) with cardiac CT geometry (CARTOSEG); panel B shows the delineation of the left pulmonary veins and the carina (*dotted yellow lines*); panel C shows the color doppler across the left inferior pulmonary vein showing flows into the LA; panel D shows the measurement of the flow velocities obtained from the left inferior pulmonary vein. LA, left atrium; LAO, left anterior oblique; LIPV, left inferior pulmonary vein; LSPV, left superior pulmonary vein.

anatomic structure, ablation on the atrial side of the veins rather within them to avoid long-term complications such as vein stenosis and achieving antral isolation.

Moreover, color and waveform doppler echocardiography is capable with ICE and can be used to record the pulmonary vein velocities[11] (see **Figs. 2** and **3**). The ability to monitor the lesion while ablating and detecting microbubbles can also help avoid complications such as steam pops even before impedance increases. Early detection of complications such as clots and pericardial effusion can avert a catastrophe.[12,13]

INTRACARDIAC ECHOCARDIOGRAPHY–GUIDED LEFT ATRIAL APPENDAGE CLOSURE

Percutaneous LAA closure with devices has evolved into a potential strategy for prophylactic stroke prevention without the need for long-term anticoagulation. Using ICE, one can appreciate a detailed delineation of the anatomy of the LAA from multiple views from the right atrium, right ventricle, LA, and even from the pulmonary artery and the coronary sinus (**Figs. 4** and **5**). Although transesophageal echocardiography is the gold standard for guidance in LAA closure, ICE is being increasingly used as an alternative.[14] ICE can be

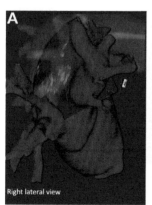
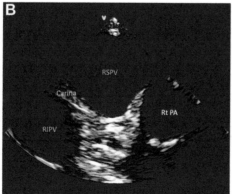
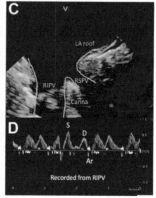

Fig. 3. *Visualization of the right pulmonary veins*: panel A shows the real-time integration of the echocardiographic section (CARTOSOUND) with cardiac CT geometry (CARTOSEG) in the right lateral view; panel B shows the short-axis view of the right pulmonary veins; panel C shows the long-axis view of the right pulmonary veins and the delineation of the right pulmonary veins and the carina (*yellow lines*); panel D shows the measurement of the flow velocities obtained from the right inferior pulmonary vein. LA, left atrium; RIPV, right inferior pulmonary vein; RSPV, right superior pulmonary vein; Rt PA, right pulmonary artery.

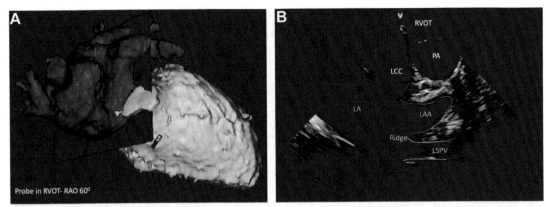

Fig. 4. *Short-axis view of the left atrial appendage*: panel A shows the real-time integration of the echocardiographic section (CARTOSOUND) with cardiac CT geometry (CARTOSEG) in the right anterior oblique (RAO) view obtained with the ICE probe in the right ventricular outflow tract (RVOT); panel B shows the short-axis view of the LAA. The ridge between the LAA and LSPV can also be appreciated. The LV summit portion of the interventricular septum with the 2 coronary vessels (red circles—left anterior descending and left circumflex) is also seen here. Note the boundaries of the LV summit. LA, left atrium; LAA, left atrial appendage; LCC, left coronary aortic cusp; LSPV, left superior pulmonary vein; PA, pulmonary artery; RVOT, right ventricular outflow tract.

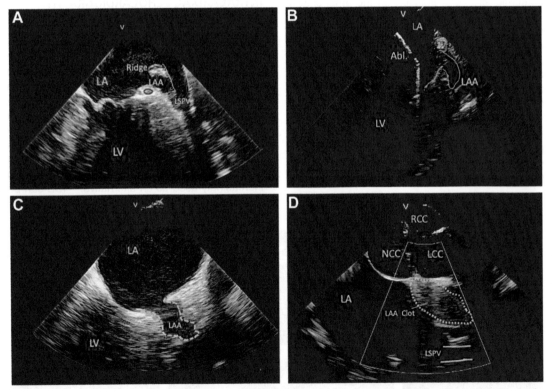

Fig. 5. *Visualization of the left atrial appendage*: panel A shows the long-axis view of the LAA obtained from the ICE probe within the LA cavity. The ridge between the LAA and the LSPV, the anterior mitral annulus, and atrioventricular groove containing the left circumflex vessel (red circle) are seen; panel B shows the long-axis view of the left atrial appendage (delineated with *yellow lines*) and the tip of the ablation catheter (Abl.) in the left atrial (LA) cavity; panel C shows the delineation of a "broccoli"-shaped LAA in its long axis obtained with the ICE probe in the right atrium; panel D shows the short-axis view obtained with the ICE probe in the right ventricle outflow, and this reveals a large soft clot filling the cavity of the LAA (delineated with *yellow lines*). LA, left atrium; LAA, left atrial appendage; LCC, left coronary aortic cusp; LSPV, left superior pulmonary vein; NCC, noncoronary aortic cusp; RCC, right coronary aortic cusp.

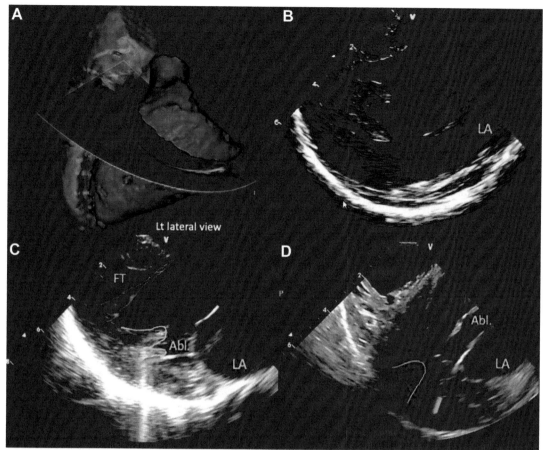

Fig. 6. *The left ventricle antero-lateral papillary muscle*: panel A shows the real-time integration of the echocardio-graphic section (CARTOSOUND) across the basal LV with cardiac CT geometry (CARTOSEG) with the ICE probe in the right ventricular outflow tract (RVOT); panel B shows the 2 heads of this "bifid" variant of anterolateral papillary muscle; panel C shows the ablation catheter (*green tip*) via transseptal access at the lateral aspect of the anterolat-eral papillary muscle. Also seen is a thick false tendon (FT) connecting the anterior wall of the left ventricle to the septum; panel D shows the ablation catheter (*green tip*) via transseptal access at the lateral basal LV.

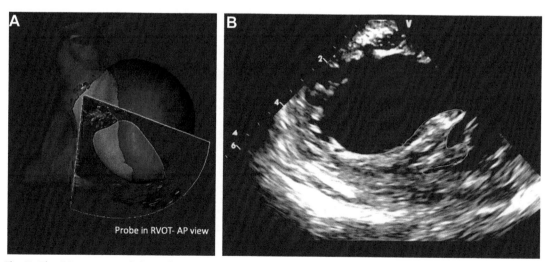

Fig. 7. *The LV posteromedial papillary muscle*: panel A shows the real-time integration of the echocardiographic section (CARTOSOUND) across the basal LV with cardiac CT geometry (CARTOSEG) in the anteroposterior (AP) view with the ICE probe in the right ventricular outflow tract (RVOT); panel B shows the attachment of the post-eromedial papillary muscle (delineated with *yellow lines*) to the posterior wall of the LV.

used as a guidance in patients in whom inducing general anesthesia or introducing an esophageal echo probe is considered difficult or risky for many reasons.

The following steps represent one form of workflow that can be adopted for LAA closure. After ruling out LAA clot, a transseptal view is obtained on the ICE probe to visualize the superoinferior extent of the atrial septum. The inferior and posterior region of the fossa ovalis is a good position to attempt puncture of the septum for LAA closure. After transseptal crossing, the ICE probe is negotiated through the puncture site into the LA. Reliable views of the morphology of the LAA, ridge between the LAA and the pulmonary vein, circumflex artery at the atrioventricular groove, and the mitral annular plane are obtained with the ICE probe within the LA. Although cardiac CT measurements are still considered the gold standard for measuring the LAA dimensions, ICE can be used to verify the dimensions of the LAA and precisely deploy the device. Device deployment is performed with continuous monitored under ICE. The operator can verify device stability, the compression of device and its relation to the left circumflex artery, and device leaks.[15] The interaction of the device with the left pulmonary vein or mitral valve can also be noted. Complications such as device embolization, compression of circumflex vessel, device leaks, pericardial effusions, and residual atrial septal defects can be monitored with ICE.[15]

ACCESSORY PATHWAY ABLATION

ICE can be used to access the LA for ablation of the left accessory pathways at the mitral annulus.

Ablation of these pathways can at times be very challenging, especially those located postero- and anteroseptally. A more anterior plane during transseptal access might be preferred for accessing structures such as the mitral annulus and basal LV. ICE helps ruling out clot before accessing the LA, ensuring contact of the ablation catheter at these locations, and monitoring for complications like pericardial effusion.[16]

ABLATION OF LEFT VENTRICULAR TACHYCARDIAS

ICE enables visualization of the LV and the intracavitary structures such as the anterolateral and posteromedial papillary muscles (**Figs. 6** and **7**). Ventricular tachycardias can originate from various regions of the LV including these intracavitary structures. For ablation of left ventricular tachycardias, although can be approached retrogradely through the aorta, certain regions of the LV such as the lateral heads of the papillary muscles, basal-lateral LV, and mitral annular ventricular tachycardias (VTs) are best approached antegradely from the LA by means of transseptal access. Although mapping for sources of VT, visualization of calcification in one of the heads of the papillary muscles or delineation of infarct zones in the LV often point toward a possible substrate.[17] Moreover, real-time imaging with ICE helps operator in ensuring continuous catheter contact with these intracavitary structures, while safely avoiding the tip of these muscles so as not to disrupt the chordae. Unfortunately, catheter contact can still be difficult and in those cases, ICE can help to ascertain that, and operator may decide to switch strategies and may use cryoablation.[18]

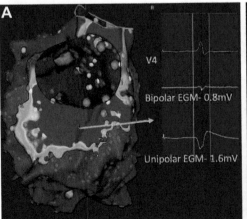
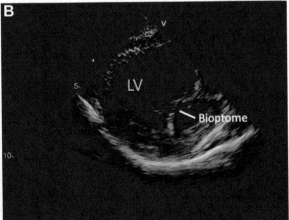

Fig. 8. *ICE-guided endomyocardial biopsy*: panel A shows the electroanatomical bipolar voltage map of LV suggesting low bipolar and unipolar voltages indicating basal lateral scar (*red zone*) in a patient with nonischemic cardiomyopathy; panel B shows the ultrasound image of the bioptome after sampling a tissue from the zone of the scar in the LV through a transseptal access.

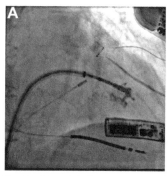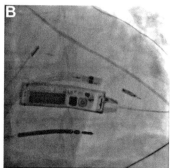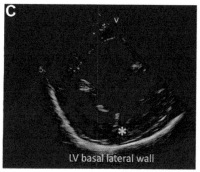

Fig. 9. *ICE-guided WiSE-CRT implant:* panel A shows the electrode delivery catheter of the WiSE-CRT system placed in the LV through transseptal route so as to access the basal lateral LV; contrast staining of the endocardial LV is also seen in the right anterior oblique view; panel B shows the wireless LV endocardial electrode deployed in the LV lateral wall; panel C shows the intracardiac echocardiography image of the endocardial electrode (asterix) in the basal lateral L.

The large curve of cryo-catheter may be difficult to prolapse in ventricle through retrograde approach. ICE-guided transeptal puncture in an anterior plane and transmitral sheath placement and use of catheter may help to achieve catheter stability. Patients with mechanical aortic valve prosthesis or hemodynamic support devices such as the Impella placed across the aortic valve would also require transseptal access in order to approach the LV and ablate arrhythmias.

NONABLATIVE ELECTROPHYSIOLOGY PROCEDURES REQUIRING TRANSSEPTAL ACCESS

Real-time integration of ICE with regions with voltage abnormalities has been explored to increase the diagnostic accuracies of endomyocardial biopsies[19] (**Fig. 8**). Live sampling of the tissues from these regions with the aid of ICE immensely add to the diagnostic and prognostic value of the biopsies. ICE also ensures in avoiding complications such as injury to the mitral valve apparatus while performing the biopsies.

Accessing the latest site of activation of the LV for placement of wireless LV endocardial leads such as the WiSE-CRT system would sometimes require transseptal access so as to better reach the targeted region and also to maintain adequate contact of the catheter against the LV endocardium while deploying the device (**Fig. 9**).

SUMMARY

Use of ICE for EP procedures has been critical in understanding the substrate anatomically along with its electrophysiological properties, more so by allowing real-time integration onto electroanatomical mapping. ICE has also superseded the

need of fluoroscopy for transseptal access or even the need of general anesthesia and transesophageal echocardiography by giving exceptional images of the interatrial septum and all of the left atrial structures. ICE has increased both the safety and efficacy of the ablations. The utility of ICE cannot be overemphasized for the visualization of the LAA, especially for deployment of LAA closure devices. Transseptal access has provided an alternate means of ablation of regions of the LV such as the papillary muscles and the basal-lateral LV, which could be source of ventricular arrhythmias. ICE is also being used for LV endocardial biopsies and for placement of LV endocardial leads. With exciting developments awaiting the technology of ICE, it will remain to stay as an indispensable tool in the armamentarium of cardiac electrophysiologists.[20]

CLINICS CARE POINTS

- ICE has enhanced the safety and efficacy of EP procedures.

- ICE-guided transseptal catherization can circumvent the need for transesophageal echocardiography and minimize the need for fluoroscopy. Transseptal catherization is an important step to access the LA and the LV.

- Monitoring of catheter contact during ablation procedures, appreciation of adjacent cardiac structures, early detection of complications, and reaching the regions of LV inaccessible via the routine aortic approach are added utilities of ICE-guided transseptal catherization.

- The plane of visualization of interatrial septum is key to plan the site of crossing the septum, as this varies depending on the procedures such as an anterior plane for pulmonary vein isolation and posterior plane for LAA closures.

- ICE is being increasingly used for integrating anatomic data onto 3-dimensional electroanatomical maps, obtaining biopsies from the LV, and placing left ventricular endocardial electrodes.

DISCLOSURES

Dr P. Sanders reports having served on the advisory board of Medtronic, Abbott Medical, Boston Scientific, CathRx, and PaceMate. Dr P. Sanders reports that the University of Adelaide has received on his behalf lecture and/or consulting fees from Medtronic, Abbott Medical, and Boston Scientific. Dr P. Sanders reports that the University of Adelaide has received on his behalf research funding from Medtronic, Abbott Medical, Boston Scientific, and Microport. All other authors have no disclosures. Dr R.K. Pathak reports having served on the advisory board of Medtronic, Abbott Medical, and Boston Scientific. Dr R.K. Pathak reports that Canberra Heart Rhythm Foundation has received on his behalf lecture and/or consulting fees from Medtronic, Abbott Medical, Boston Scientific, and Biotronik. Dr R.K. Pathak reports that Canberra Heart Rhythm Foundation has received on his behalf research funding from Medtronic, Abbott Medical, Boston Scientific, and Biotronik.

ACKNOWLEDGMENTS

Dr P. Sanders is supported by a Practitioner Fellowship from the National Health and Medical Research Council of Australia and by the National Heart Foundation of Australia.

REFERENCES

1. Hijazi ZM, Shivkumar K, Sahn DJ. Intracardiac echocardiography during interventional and electrophysiological cardiac catheterization. Circulation 2009; 119:587–96.
2. Enriquez A, Saenz LC, Rosso R, et al. Use of intracardiac echocardiography in interventional Cardiology. Circulation 2018;137(21):2278–94.
3. Razminia M, Willoughby MC, Demo H, et al. Fluoroless catheter ablation of cardiac arrhythmias: a 5-year experience. Pacing Clin Electrophysiol 2017; 40:425–33.
4. Reddy VY, Neuzil P, Koruth JS, et al. Pulsed field ablation for pulmonary vein isolation in atrial fibrillation. J Am Coll Cardiol 2019;74(3):315–26.
5. Calkins H, Hindricks G, Cappato R, et al. 2017HRS/EHRA/ECAS/APHRS/SOLAECE expert consensus statement on catheter andsurgical ablation of atrial fibrillation. Heart Rhythm 2017; 14:e275–444.
6. Verma A, Jiang C, Betts TR, et al. Approaches to catheter ablation for persistent atrial fibrillation. N Engl J Med 2015;372:1812–22.
7. Marrouche NF, Martin DO, Wazni O, et al. Phased-array intracardiac echocardiography monitoring during pulmonary vein isolation in patients with atrial fibrillation: impact on outcome and complications. Circulation 2003;107:2710–6.
8. Hsu JC, Badhwar N, Gerstenfeld EP, et al. Randomized trial of conventional transseptal needle versus radiofrequency energy needle puncture for left atrial access (the TRAVERSE-LA study). J Am Heart Assoc 2013;2:e000428.
9. Lakkireddy D, Rangisetty U, Prasad S, et al. Intracardiac echo-guided radiofrequency catheter ablation of atrial fibrillation in patients with atrial septal defect or patent foramen ovale repair: a feasibility, safety, and efficacy study. J Cardiovasc Electrophysiol 2008;19:1137–42.
10. Santangeli P, Di Biase L, Burkhardt JD, et al. Transseptal access and atrial fibrillation ablation guided by intracardiac echocardiography in patients with atrial septal closure devices. Heart Rhythm 2011;8: 1669–75.
11. Ren JF, Marchlinski FE, Callans DJ, et al. Intracardiac Doppler echocardiographic quantification of pulmonary vein flow velocity: an effective technique for monitoring pulmonary vein ostia narrowing during focal atrial fibrillation ablation. J Cardiovasc Electrophysiol 2002;13:1076–108.
12. Cury RC, Abbara S, Schmidt S, et al. Relationship of the esophagus and aorta to the left atrium and pulmonary veins: implications for catheter ablation of atrial fibrillation. Heart Rhythm 2005; 2:1317–23.
13. Ren JF, Callans DJ, Schwartzman D, et al. Changes in local wall thickness correlate with pathologic lesion size following radiofrequency catheter ablation: an intracardiac echocardiographic imaging study. Echocardiography 2001;18:503–7.
14. Alkhouli M, Chaker Z, Alqahtani F, et al. Outcomes of routine intracardiac echocardiography to Guide left atrial appendage occlusion. JACC Clin Electrophysiol 2020;6(4):393–400.
15. Paiva LV, Costa MP, Barra SC, et al. Intracardiac echography for left atrial appendage closure: a step-by-step tutorial. Catheter Cardiovasc Interv 2019;93(5):e302–10.
16. West JJ, Norton PT, Kramer CM, et al. Characterization of the mitral isthmus for atrial fibrillation ablation using intracardiac ultrasound from within the coronary sinus. Heart Rhythm 2008;5:19–27.

17. Enriquez A, Supple GE, Marchlinski FE, et al. How to map and ablate papillary muscle ventricular arrhythmias. Heart Rhythm 2017;14:1721–8.

18. Gordon JP, Liang JJ, Pathak RK, et al. Percutaneous cryoablation for papillary muscle ventricular arrhythmias after failed radiofrequency catheter ablation. J Cardiovasc Electrophysiol 2018;29(12): 1654–63.

19. Casella M, Dello Russo A, Vettor G, et al. Electroanatomical mapping systems and intracardiac echo integration for guided endomyocardial biopsy. Expert Rev Med Devices 2017;14:609–19.

20. Khuri-Yakub BT, Oralkan O. Capacitive micromachined ultrasonic transducers for medical imaging and therapy. J Micromech Microeng 2011;21: 54004–14.

Intracardiac Echocardiography to Guide Catheter Ablation of Atrial Fibrillation

Carola Gianni, MD[a],*, Javier E. Sanchez, MD[a],
Domenico G. Della Rocca, MD[a], Amin Al-Ahmad, MD[a],
Rodney P. Horton, MD[a], Luigi Di Biase, MD[a,b], Andrea Natale, MD[a,c,d,e]

KEYWORDS

• Intracardiac echocardiography • Atrial fibrillation ablation • Atrial fibrillation ablation complications

KEY POINTS

• Intracardiac echocardiography (ICE) allows for real-time assessment of cardiac anatomy.
• ICE has many different applications during atrial fibrillation ablation procedures, allowing limiting radiation exposure to the patient and staff, identifying relevant anatomic structures, facilitating transseptal access, assessing accurate placement (including contact) of mapping and ablation catheters, and recognizing complications early.
• A baseline cardiac survey with ICE is useful to quantify baseline pericardial effusion as well as rule out left atrial appendage thrombosis.

INTRODUCTION

Intracardiac echocardiography (ICE) is an invaluable tool in electrophysiology. ICE provides real-time bi-dimensional ultrasound imaging obtained by phased-array transducers, allowing for real-time assessment of cardiac anatomy as well as procedure guidance and complications' monitoring. More specifically, during atrial fibrillation, ICE is used throughout the procedure with a variety of applications, including (but not limited to)

• Limiting radiation exposure to the patient and staff[1]
• Identifying relevant anatomic structures

• Facilitating transseptal access
• assessing accurate placement (including contact) of mapping and ablation catheters
• Recognizing complications early

In this short overview, we will describe our approach in using real-time ICE imaging during atrial fibrillation (AF) ablation procedures.

PROCEDURE GUIDANCE
Baseline Cardiac Survey

At the beginning of the procedure, we perform a basic cardiac ultrasound survey with ICE to identify abnormal/challenging anatomy (such as, left common os, accessory pulmonary veins [PVs], or

No relevant conflicts of interest to disclose.
All the authors share the same contact information as the corresponding author.
Funding: none.
[a] Texas Cardiac Arrhythmia Institute, St. David's Medical Center, Austin, TX, USA; [b] Montefiore Medical Center, Bronx, NY, USA; [c] HCA National Medical Director of Cardiac Electrophysiology, Nashville, TN, USA; [d] Interventional Electrophysiology, Scripps Clinic, La Jolla, CA, USA; [e] MetroHealth Medical Center, Case Western Reserve University School of Medicine, Cleveland, OH, USA
* Corresponding author.
E-mail address: carola.gianni@gmail.com

Card Electrophysiol Clin 13 (2021) 303–311
https://doi.org/10.1016/j.ccep.2021.03.009

left persistent superior vena cava [LPSVC];) and quantify baseline pericardial fluid. By positioning the ICE catheter in the right atrium (RA) and right ventricle (RV), we obtain the following views:

- ICE in the RA (**Fig. 1**)
  1. The catheter is positioned it the mid-RA, in a neutral position, showing the "home view" (see below)
  2. With sequential clockwise rotation
     a. Home view, ie, cavo-tricuspid isthmus (CTI) and tricuspid valve (TV)
     b. RV outflow tract (RVOT), aortic root and valve (with the non-coronary cusp being the closest cusp to the RA), and pulmonary valve and artery
     c. Coronary sinus (CS) ostium
     d. Left ventricle (LV), anterior interatrial septum (IAS), mitral valve, left atrial appendage (LAA)
     e. Mid-IAS, descending aorta/esophagus, left PVs
     f. Posterior IAS, esophagus
     g. Right PVs, pulmonary artery
     h. Posterior RA, superior vena cava (SVC)
     i. Crista terminalis, RA appendage (RAA)
- ICE in the RV (**Fig. 2**)
  1. From the RA, the catheter is deflected anteriorly when visualizing the RAA, advanced past the TV leaflets, and undeflected in a neutral position (like this, the catheter lies in the basal RVOT).
     a. It is important not to rely on fluoroscopy for this maneuver, as the heart rotation is variable with a non-negligible risk of perforation when advancing the stiff ICE probe.
  2. With sequential clockwise rotation
     a. Initial view: RV, moderator band
     b. Interventricular septum
     c. LV (inferior and anterior wall), inferoseptal papillary muscle (PM)
     d. LV (septal and lateral wall), mitral valve (MV), antero-lateral PM, LV outflow tract
     e. Left superior PV, ridge, LAA
     f. Aortic cusps (short axis, with the right coronary cusp closest to the RV and left coronary cusp farthest), left main and proximal left anterior descending/circumflex coronary artery, posterior RVOT
     g. Mid and anterior RVOT, pulmonary valve and artery
     h. Aortic root (long axis), right coronary artery
     i. SVC

Left Atrial Appendage Thrombus

Of note, before trans-septal access, the LAA is visualized carefully with the ICE catheter positioned in the RA and the basal RVOT (discussed previously) to rule out LAA thrombosis (**Fig. 3**).[2–5] When the ICE catheter is positioned in the RVOT, small movements of the tip of the ICE catheter (lateral-medial deflection vs advancing and retracting, according to the specific LAA morphology) are necessary to visualize the full body of the LAA (from the ostium to the tip).

Trans-septal Access

ICE also is an invaluable tool to perform trans-septal access:

- Uncomplicated LA access is confirmed by real-time visualization of the needle tenting and passing the IAS along with bubbles in the LA when injecting saline through the needle (**Fig. 4**).
  1. As such, when using ICE, pressure monitoring and contrast injection are superfluous.
- LA access can be obtained safely also with otherwise challenging anatomical variants (ie, lipomatous or aneurysmatic septum) and prior atrial septal defect closure[6] (**Fig. 5**).
- To facilitate PV isolation, transseptal access should be
  1. Posterior for radiofrequency (RF) ablation, ie, through the IAS when the left PVs or the posterior wall next to them are in view (see **Fig. 4**)
  2. Mid-IAS for cryoablation, ie, through the IAS when the left PVs or left PVs/LAA ridge is in view (the mitral valve should not be visible, because it would denote a too anterior stick)

Mapping and Ablation

During mapping and ablation, we mainly use ICE to guide proper catheter positioning:

- For PV isolation, antral location of the circular mapping and ablation catheters as well as of cryo- and RF- ablation balloons (**Fig. 6**)
  1. As stated above, ICE also allows to idenfity PV anatomical variants (**Fig. 7**).
- For LAA isolation, the catheters are positioned at the level of the ostium (see **Fig. 6**), and not deeper, to minimize the risk of perforation and phrenic nerve paralysis during ablation.[7]
- For CS isolation, ICE allows to easily cannulate the CS by visualizing its ostium and

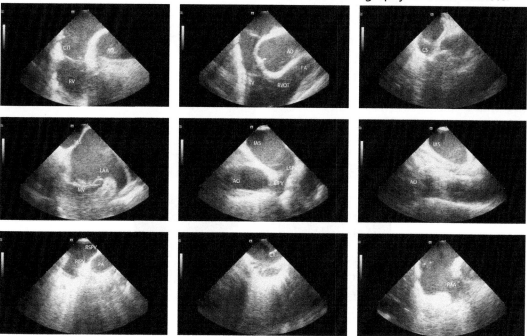

Fig. 1. Cardiac survey with the ICE probe in the RA. See relative text for description. AO, aorta; CS, coronary sinus; CT, crista terminalis; CTI, cavo-tricuspid isthmus; Eso, esophagus; IAS, interatrial septum; ICE, intracardiac echocardiography; LAA, left atrial appendage; LIPV, left inferior pulmonary vein; LSPV, left superior pulmonary vein; MV, mitral valve; RA, right atrium; RAA, right atrial appendage; RIPV, right inferior pulmonary vein; RSPV, right superior pulmonary vein; RV, right ventricle; RVOT, right ventricular outflow tract.

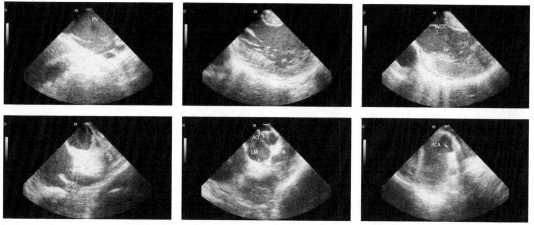

Fig. 2. Cardiac survey with the ICE probe in the RV. See relative text for description. alPM, antero-lateral papillary muscle; AO, aorta; ICE, intracardiac echocardiography; isPM, septal papillary muscle; LAA, left atrial appendage; LM, left main coronary artery; LSPV, left superior pulmonary vein; MB, moderator band; RCA, right coronary artery; RV, right ventricle.

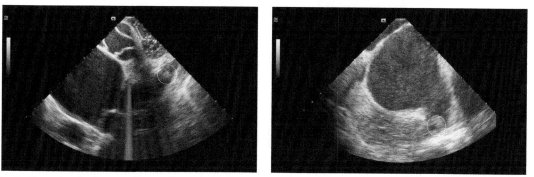

Fig. 3. Thrombus in the LAA detected with ICE before transseptal access. (*Left*) View obtained from the RV; (*right*) view obtained from the RA.

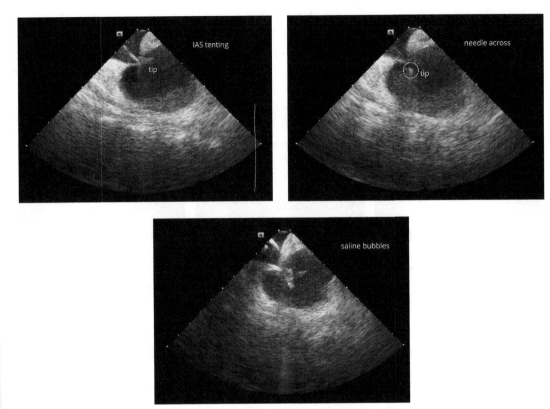

Fig. 4. ICE-guided trans-septal access. See relative text for description.

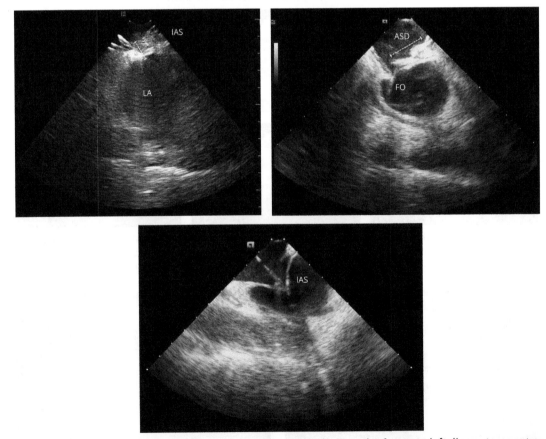

Fig. 5. Examples of difficult transseptal access anatomies. In clockwise order from top left: lipomatous septum, aneurysmatic septum, and ASD closure device. ASD, atrial septal defect; FO, fossa ovalis; LA, left atrium.

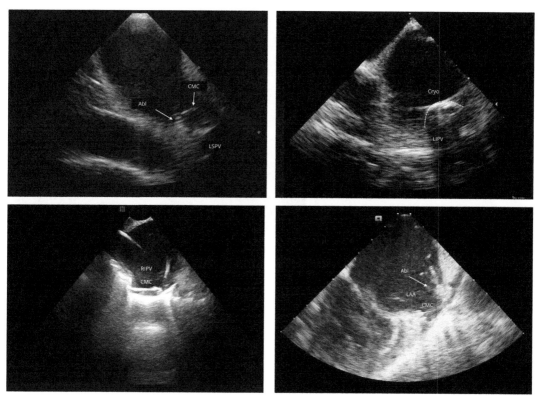

Fig. 6. ICE for PV and LAA isolation. Abl, ablation catheter; CMC, circular mapping catheter; Cryo, cryoballoon catheter; LAA, left atrial appendage; LIPV, left inferior pulmonary vein; LSPV, left superior pulmonary vein; RIPV, right inferior pulmonary vein. Adapted with permission from Cardiotext Publishing.[8] (Gianni C, Perez MV, Al-Ahmad A, Natale A. How to perform pulmonary vein antral isolation for atrial fibrillation. In: Hands-On Ablation: The Experts' Approach Al-Ahmad A, Callans DJ, Hsia HH, Natale A, Oseroff O, Wang PJ (editors). Second edition. Cardiotext; 2017. p. 135 to 144.).

facilitates its complete isolation by visualizing its endocardial aspect to be targeted with ablation[7] (**Fig. 8**).

- For SVC isolation, ICE is used to identify the junction between the RA and SVC, which lies across the area between the ostium of the right superior PV and right pulmonary artery (**Fig. 9**).

- For LPSVC isolation, the circular mapping catheter can be visualized inside the dilated CS and moved under ultrasound guidance (**Fig. 10**).

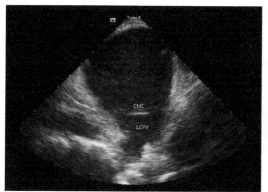
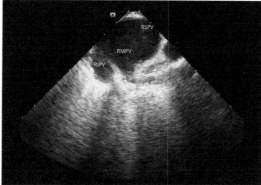

Fig. 7. PV anatomical variants. (*Left*) Common os for the left PVs; (*right*) right middle PV. CMC, circular mapping catheter; LCPV, left common PV; RIPM, right inferior pulmonary vein; RMPV, right middle PV; RSPV, right superior PV.

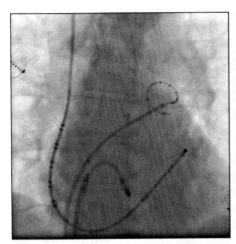
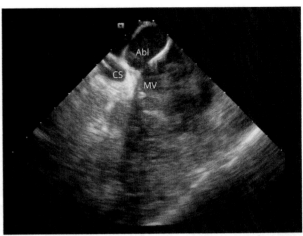

Fig. 8. ICE for CS isolation. Abl, ablation catheter; CS, coronary sinus; MV, mitral valve.

- For CTI-dependent atrial flutter ablation (**Fig. 11**), the patient's specific CTI anatomy can be easily delineated, which is especially important in repeat procedures or when bi-directional block is hard to achieve.
    1. A prominent eustachian ridge and pouches easily are visualized and can be navigated with the ablation catheter in real time.

During RF energy delivery, ICE can be used to visualize the tip of the ablation catheter and confirm proper tissue-catheter contact throughout the cardiac cycle, even when not using contact force–sensing catheters. ICE can also be used to monitor for tissue overheating (ie, excessive hyperechogenicity on ICE) and prevent subsequent steam pops.

Another important application of ICE is the delineation of the course of the esophagus in real time,

limiting RF application on top of it (**Fig. 12**). Of note, the location of an esophageal temperature probe on fluoroscopy is not a good indicator of esophageal course, as the esophagus is wider than the probe itself.

COMPLICATIONS MONITORING

Finally, ICE is vital to monitor for complications and identify their etiology, allowing for early intervention:

- Unexpected hypotension: ICE can quickly rule out devastating vascular complications (eg, aortic dissection, retroperitoneal hematoma) and significant pericardial effusion (increased volume from baseline).
    1. With ICE in the iliac vein and inferior vena cava, it is possible to visualize the retroperitoneal space and the presence of

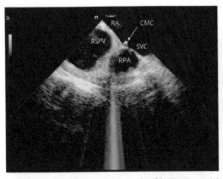
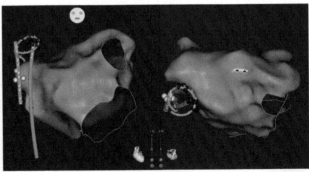

Fig. 9. ICE for SVC isolation. (*Left*) CMC positioned in the SVC-RA junction, which corresponds to area between the RSPV ostium and right pulmonary artery; (*right*) SVC isolation obtained by segmental isolation at the level of the SVC-RA junction. CMC, circular mapping catheter; RA, right atrium atrium; RPA, right pulmonary artery; RSPV, right superior pulmonary vein; SVC, superior vena cava. (Adapted with permission from Oxford University Press.[7]). (Gianni C, Mohanty S, Trivedi C, Di Biase L, Natale A. Novel concepts and approaches in ablation of atrial fibrillation: the role of non-pulmonary vein triggers. EP Eur. 2018 Oct 1;20(10):1566–76.)

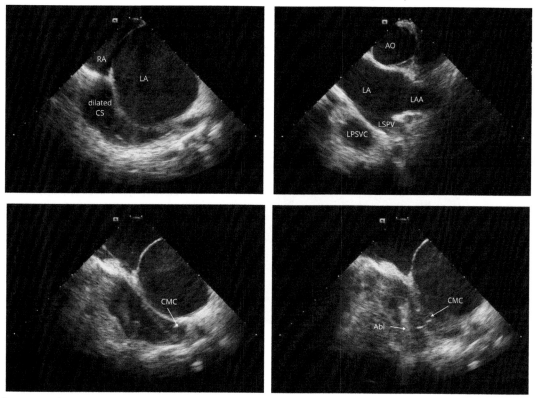

Fig. 10. ICE for LPSVC isolation. (*Top*) Anatomic features in case of LPSVC. (*Bottom*) CMC inside the dilated CS (distal and mid) during LSPVC isolation. Abl, ablation catheter; AO, aorta; CMC, circular mapping catheter; CS, coronary sinus; LA, left atrium; LAA, left atrial appendage; LPSVC, left persistent superior vena cava; LSPV, left superior pulmonary vein; RA, right atrium.

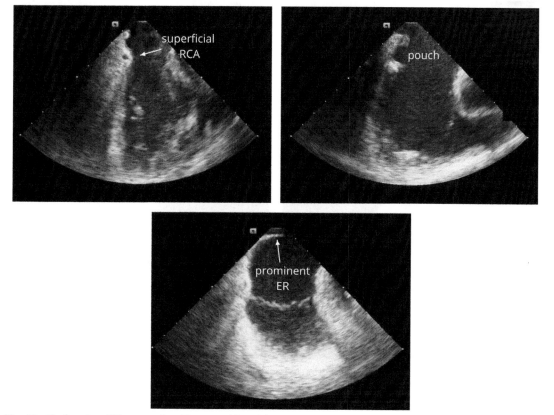

Fig. 11. Challenging CTI anatomies. ER, eustachian ridge; RCA, right coronary artery.

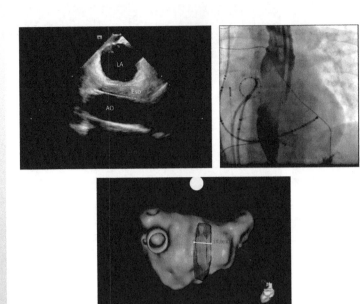

Fig. 12. Esophageal course on ICE. Abl, ablation catheter; AO, aorta; CMC, circular mapping catheter; LA, left atrium; LSPV, left superior PV. AO, aorta; Eso, esophagus; LA, left atrium. (Adapted with permission from John Wiley and Sons.[9] (Gianni C, Della Rocca DG, MacDonald BC, Mohanty S, Quintero Mayedo A, Sahore Salwan A, et al. Prevention, diagnosis, and management of atrioesophageal fistula. Pacing Clin Electrophysiol. 2020 Jul;43(7):640–5.))

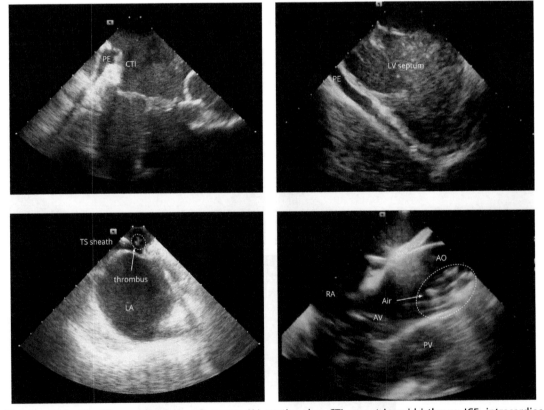

Fig. 13. ICE to identify complications. AO, aorta; AV, aortic valve; CTI, cavo-tricuspid isthmus; ICE, intracardiac echocardiography; LA, left atrium; LV, left ventricle; PE, pericardial effusion; PV, pulmonary valve; RA, right atrium; TS, trans-septal.

hematoma (a heterogeneously echoic mass; acutely, it is composed of small moving speckles, representing active bleeding with partial thrombus formation) and the abdominal aorta and the presence of a false lumen.

2. Initially, pericardial effusion is typically seen behind the CTI (RA view **Fig. 13**); and at the level of the atrio-ventricular groove behind the MV (RV view); in the absence of adhesions, in a prone patient, additional fluid accumulates around the RV and LV (see **Fig. 13**).

- ST segment changes
  1. ST depression is usually secondary to demand ischemia: with ICE, calcium can be seen in the aorta/ostium of the right/left main coronary artery and it is possible to observe a transient decrease in regional/global LV function.
     a. When calcium is observed at the level of the coronary arteries, the authors limit the dose of isoproterenol/dobutamine during drug challenge.
  2. ST elevation is a more serious complication: it is important to look for thrombus formation over the sheath/catheters or presence of aortic air embolism (see **Fig. 13**).
     a. It is important to recognize the etiology guide the proper intervention (ie, anticoagulation/thrombolysis, percutaneous coronary intervention vs air aspiration, and pressure support).

CLINICS CARE POINTS

- In the spirit of ALARA (as low as reasonably achievable), ICE is a valuable tool to limit radiation exposure to the patient and staff.
- ICE enhances the operator's knowledge of the patient's specific anatomy and relevant anatomic variations.
- Transseptal puncture performed under real-time ICE guidance allows for quick, safe, and precise left atrial access.
- Catheters can be visualized with ICE during the procedure and their placement (including contact with tissue) can be accurately assessed to guide mapping and ablation.
- ICE allows for continuous monitoring of many AF ablation-related complications, such as pericardial effusion, catheter-/sheath-related

thrombosis, or air embolism, leading to early recognition and treatment.

REFERENCES

1. Razminia M, Zei PC, editors. Fluoroscopy reduction techniques for catheter ablation of cardiac arrhythmias. First edition. Minneapolis, Missouri, USA: Cardiotext; 2019. .

2. Baran J, Stec S, Pilichowska-Paszkiet E, et al. Intracardiac echocardiography for detection of thrombus in the left atrial appendage comparison with transesophageal echocardiography in patients undergoing ablation for atrial fibrillation: the Action-ICE I study. Circ Arrhythm Electrophysiol 2013;6(6):1074–81.

3. Di Biase L, Briceno DF, Trivedi C, et al. Is transesophageal echocardiogram mandatory in patients undergoing ablation of atrial fibrillation with uninterrupted novel oral anticoagulants? Results from a prospective multicenter registry. Heart Rhythm 2016;13(6):1197–202.

4. Baran J, Zaborska B, Piotrowski R, et al. Intracardiac echocardiography for verification for left atrial appendage thrombus presence detected by transesophageal echocardiography: the Action-ICE II study. Clin Cardiol 2017;40(7):450–4.

5. Patel K, Natale A, Yang R, et al. Is transesophageal echocardiography necessary in patients undergoing ablation of atrial fibrillation on an uninterrupted direct oral anticoagulant regimen? Results from a prospective multicenter registry. Heart Rhythm 2020;17(12):2093–9.

6. Lakkireddy D, Rangisetty U, Prasad S, et al. Intracardiac echo-guided radiofrequency catheter ablation of atrial fibrillation in patients with atrial septal defect or patent foramen Ovale repair: a feasibility, safety, and efficacy study. J Cardiovasc Electrophysiol 2008;19(11):1137–42.

7. Gianni C, Mohanty S, Trivedi C, et al. Novel concepts and approaches in ablation of atrial fibrillation: the role of non-pulmonary vein triggers. Europace 2018;20(10):1566–76.

8. Gianni C, Perez MV, Al-Ahmad A, et al. How to perform pulmonary vein antral isolation for atrial fibrillation. In: Al-Ahmad A, Callans DJ, Hsia HH, et al, editors. Hands-on ablation: the Experts' approach. Second edition. Minneapolis, Missouri, USA: Cardiotext; 2017. p. 135–44.

9. Gianni C, Della Rocca DG, MacDonald BC, et al. Prevention, diagnosis, and management of atrioesophageal fistula. Pacing Clin Electrophysiol 2020;43(7):640–5.

Role of Intracardiac Echography for Transcatheter Occlusion of Left Atrial Appendage

Apoor Patel, MD, Miguel Valderrábano, MD*

KEYWORDS

- Left atrial appendage occlusion • Watchman • Amplatzer • Intracardiac echocardiography
- Transesophageal echocardiogram

KEY POINTS

- Intracardiac echocardiogram can be used safely for all aspects of left atrial appendage occlusion, including transseptal puncture, appendage ostial measurements, sheath insertion, and assessment of device release criteria.
- Appendage occlusion under intracardiac echocardiography has shown similar implant efficacy and safety compared with transesophageal echocardiography in nonrandomized studies.
- General or deep anesthesia can be avoided with an intracardiac echocardiography–guided strategy.
- Total in-room time and turnaround time are faster with an intracardiac echocardiography–guided strategy, and global hospital costs are not increased compared with transesophageal echocardiography.
- With intracardiac echocardiography from the left atrium, 3 main views of the left atrial appendage facilitate device deployment and assessment. The authors recommend a home view from the mid-left atrium, a view from the left superior pulmonary vein, and a view from the mitral annulus.

INTRODUCTION

Left atrial appendage closure (LAAC) is an increasingly common procedure for patients with nonvalvular atrial fibrillation (AF) and contraindications to long-term anticoagulation. Currently used closure devices include the Watchman (Boston Scientific, Natick, Massachusetts), Amplatzer Amulet (Abbott, Minneapolis, Minnesota), and Lariat (SentreHeart, Redwood City, California), with multiple other devices under investigation. In the randomized trials leading to Food and Drug Administration (FDA) approval, Watchman implantation was performed under transesophageal echocardiography (TEE) guidance.[1] Although most operators have become experienced and comfortable with TEE-guided appendage closure, there has been a growing interest in the use of intracardiac echocardiography

Funding and Conflicts of Interest: Dr M. Valderrábano is funded by NIH/NHLBI grant RO1 HL 115003; and the Charles Burnett III and Lois and Carl Davis endowments.
Conflicts of interest for all authors: None.
Division of Cardiac Electrophysiology, Department of Cardiology, Houston Methodist DeBakey Heart and Vascular Center, Houston Methodist Hospital, Houston, TX, USA
* Corresponding author. Department of Cardiology, Houston Methodist Hospital, 6550 Fannin Street, Suite 1901, Houston, TX 77030.
E-mail address: mvalderrabano@houstonmethodist.org

cardiacEP.theclinics.com

(ICE) for LAAC. This article describes the rationale and technique for ICE-guided LAAC.

CLINICAL TRIALS FOR LEFT ATRIAL APPENDAGE CLOSURE

The Watchman was FDA approved in 2015 and is the most studied LAAC device to date. The PROTECT-AF and PREVAIL trials randomized patients 2:1 to the Watchman or warfarin in patients with AF and risk for stroke. The Watchman was noninferior for the composite endpoint of all-cause stroke, systemic embolism, and death.[1,2] Longer-term results demonstrated that the Watchman arm had a significant reduction in intracranial hemorrhage as well as cardiovascular/unexplained death.[3] Registry and real-world studies confirmed a high implant success rate (>95%) with a less than 2% acute complication rate.[4] Given that direct anticoagulants are superior to warfarin with regard to hemorrhagic stroke, fatal bleeding, and mortality,[5,6] there has been significant interest in comparison of LAAC devices to direct anticoagulants. In the PRAGUE-17 trial, 402 patients with AF and either prior bleeding, embolic event while on a direct anticoagulant or a combination of high stroke and bleeding risk were randomized to LAAC (Amulet or Watchman) or direct anticoagulants (predominantly apixaban).[7] They found that LAAC was noninferior for the primary combined endpoint of AF-related cardiovascular, neurologic, and bleeding events. To further address the utility of LAAC the CHAMPION-AF trial will randomize patients to Watchman FLX or direct anticoagulants in a broader population than PRAGUE-17 (one that is able to tolerate long-term anticoagulant use).

The Amplatzer Amulet, which has CE mark approval and is available in Europe, consists of a lobe and disk connected by a flexible waist. Prospective registry data have shown a high implant success rate of greater than 99%, with an approximately 4% risk of stroke, embolism, and vascular complications within 7 days of implant.[8] The Amplatzer Amulet will be compared with direct anticoagulants in the CATALYST trial, which plans to randomize 2650 patients with embolic and bleeding–related primary endpoints. Indications for LAAC also may expand based on results of other ongoing trials, such as ASAP-TOO (antiplatelet therapy instead of oral anticoagulation immediately post Watchman implantation) and OPTION (patients undergoing ablation randomized to Watchman FLX or direct anticoagulant). In addition, as the incidence of AF increases[9,10] it is anticipated LAAC procedures will continue to grow.

ADVANTAGES OF INTRACARDIAC ECHOCARDIOGRAPHY VERSUS TRANSESOPHAGEAL ECHOCARDIOGRAPHY FOR LEFT ATRIAL APPENDAGE CLOSURE

Although TEE often is a familiar imaging modality for many cardiologists, its use is associated with disadvantages, such as the need for general anesthesia and an additional anesthesiologist or cardiologist to perform the TEE. TEE use requires more preprocedural coordination and introduces procedural inefficiencies. In this context, there has been a growing interesting in the use of ICE for LAAC placement. A majority of operators currently use phased-array ICE (compared with radial or rotational ICE). Phased-array ICE has a 64-element transducer on an 8F to 10F sheath. It allows combinations of right, left, anterior, and posterior deflection along with clockwise and counterclockwise rotation and it is able to perform Doppler and color flow imaging. ICE can guide most aspects of appendage closure, including assessment of left atrial appendage (LAA) thrombus, transseptal puncture, measurement of appendage ostium for device sizing, confirmation of delivery sheath in the appendage, and assessment of release criteria, including stability (pull), color flow for leaks, and compression measurements. In addition, it allows for monitoring of pericardial effusion throughout the procedure.

Several studies have assessed the role of TEE versus ICE for LAAC.[11–16] Hemam and colleagues[11] compared 53 patients with an ICE-guided Watchman implant strategy to 51 patients with TEE-guided implant. They found that patients with an ICE-guided implant demonstrated shorter total in-room time, turnaround time, and fluoroscopy time compared with TEE. There was 100% implant success in both groups and no differences in periprocedural complications or significant postprocedure leaks. A subsequent study studied 286 consecutively enrolled patients (90 ICE and 196 TEE) also found high implant success (>95%) in both groups with similar complication rates (<4%).[12] Follow-up imaging showed similar rates of peridevice leaks, device thrombi, and residual atrial septal defects. A multicenter Italian study assessed 187 Amplatzer devices implanted under ICE guidance compared with 417 implanted via TEE and found similar procedural success and safety between the 2 modalities.[14] They specifically looked at the complication rate of patients in the ICE group who had preprocedural CT. They found these patients had less fluoroscopy use, fewer pericardial effusions, and less need for a second device compared with patients without a CT, demonstrating the utility of preprocedural planning in LAAC. A meta-analysis of Watchman and Amulet implantation using an ICE-guided versus TEE-guided strategy found no difference in acute procedural success, procedure time, and complications, including tamponade, device embolization, and stroke, between the 2 strategies.[15] **Table 1** summarizes the advantages and disadvantages of a TEE-guided versus ICE-guided approach.

EXPENDITURES FOR INTRACARDIAC ECHOCARDIOGRAPHY–GUIDED LEFT ATRIAL APPENDAGE CLOSURE VERSUS TRANSESOPHAGEAL ECHOCARDIOGRAPHY

In an era of constantly increasing health care expenditures, and in an interventional specialty where rapid evolving technology is fundamental to the field, cost and efficiency are of particular concern. In an ICE-guided strategy there are no anesthesia fees but fees associated with the catheter, ICE technical fees, and moderate sedation charges. In the TEE group, there are TEE and anesthesia technical fees, anesthesia professional fees, and recovery room charges. Hemam and colleagues[11] found that although total hospital charges were similar between ICE and TEE, professional fees were lower in the ICE group due to a lack of anesthesia staff charges. In addition, global charges (hospital costs + professional fees) were lower in the ICE group. Alkhouli and colleagues[12] similarly found lower professional charges in the TEE group but higher hospital charges in the ICE group and equivalent global charges. Thus, overall use of ICE likely is cost-neutral with regard to global charges without accounting for the increase in efficiency that ICE confers.

ADAPTING TO AN INTRACARDIAC ECHOCARDIOGRAPHY–GUIDED IMPLANT STRATEGY

TEE-guided placement relies on 4 major views to confirm the position, seal, and compression of the device. These views are obtained with the TEE probe at the midesophageal level in the 0°, 45°, 90°, and 135° planes. The 0° view images via the horizonal (transverse) plane through the appendage whereas the 90° view images via the vertical (sagittal) plane. Ideally position, compression, and color Doppler for leak assessment are performed in all 4 views; however, there is variability in the quality of the views among operators. Adequate compression for the Watchman 2.5 device is defined as 8% to 20% and as 10% to 30% for Watchman FLX. The device may seem satisfactory in 1 view and yet not meet criteria for release in another due to inadequate compression, an overhanging device edge (shoulder) due to asymmetric deployment, or significant flow around the device into the appendage. No single view can be considered as an independent confirmation or denial of proper device deployment. Furthermore, echocardiographic views need validation with contrast angiography.

Although it seems intuitive to try to mimic the 4 TEE views when first starting with an ICE-guided approach, it is more realistic to adopt the ICE images as their own set of unique views. With proper manipulation of the ICE catheter in the left atrium (LA), a thorough assessment of the Watchman position is able to be obtained without the need to specifically mimic the 4 major TEE views. The focus should be on complementary and orthogonal views to fully assess device position. The ICE views are only approximations of TEE views

Table 1
Comparison of intracardiac echocardiography–guided versus transesophageal echocardiography–guided left atrial appendage closure implantation

	Transesophageal Echocardiography	Intracardiac Echocardiography
Advantages	High resolution Familiar imaging modality for most cardiologists Allows 3-D visualization	Familiar imaging for most electrophysiologists Reduces need for anesthesiologist Shorter procedural in-room time and turnaround time Lower professional fees
Disadvantages	Imaging quality often operator dependent Requires presence of anesthesia staff Risks of general anesthesia Risk of TEE, including esophageal and throat injury	Limitations in ability to maneuver catheter Requires dilation of transseptal or additional transseptal Additional access sheath required

because the ICE catheter has limited range of motion, has single plane imaging, and is imaging from a different vantage point than the TEE probe. Despite the limitation of ICE-based imaging, no patients required conversion to general anesthesia due to imaging concerns in studies comparing ICE and TEE.[12] IAlthough different ICE views were used among studies, they all demonstrated that ICE-based imaging is sufficient to assess device position, stability, and compression without replication of standard TEE-based multiplanar views.[11–15] Integral to the procedure, as with TEE, is the use of contrast fluoroscopy.

PREPROCEDURAL IMAGING AND ASSESSMENT OF LEFT ATRIAL APPENDAGE THROMBUS

Although not mandatory, preprocedural imaging is useful to the assess anatomy of the LAA as well as the presence of thrombus. This is important especially in high-risk patients who have a prior appendage thrombus or in patients with high burdens of AF who have not been anticoagulated prior to the procedure. The authors obtain either a TEE within 48 hours or, for patients in whom TEE cannot be performed (those with esophageal strictures, varices, and so forth), a CT with delayed imaging protocols to opacify the LAA.[17] CT has high sensitivity (>95%) and specificity (>92%) for thrombus assessment.[18,19] CT has the additional benefit of clear delineation of appendage morphology (chicken wing, windsock, cactus, or cauliflower) as well as ostial width, ostial eccentricity, and the depth of the various lobes.[20] CT use preprocedure can reduce procedure times and complications.[21] In addition, software platforms, such as 3mensio (Pie Medical Imaging, Maastricht, The Netherlands), are now available, which analyze CT images and allow 3-dimensional (3-D) manipulation to help plan device sizing, identify optimal transseptal sites, and recommend fluoroscopic views to maximize the long-axis view of the appendage during contrast angiography. Identification of certain appendage morphologies, such as a wide but shallow appendage, can have implications for the type of LAAC closure device used.

Intraprocedurally, a preliminary assessment of the LAA for the presence of thrombus can be performed using a view from the right ventricular outflow tract[22,23] and again once the ICE catheter is in the LA. The combination of views is sufficient to rule out thrombus in patients who have not had preprocedure TEE or CT. ICE surveillance of the LAA then is complemented with imaging from the RA and right ventricle to assess for the presence of baseline pericardial effusion.

OBTAINING VASCULAR ACCESS AND CHOOSING AN INTRACARDIAC ECHOCARDIOGRAPHY PROBE

The first procedural consequence of using ICE-guided LAAC is the need for an additional femoral vein puncture. Depending on the ICE probe used, either an 8F or 10F sheath is required. Available ICE probes include 8F or 10F AcuNav (Biosense Webster, Irvine, California) or 10F ViewFlex Plus (Abbott). The authors puncture the femoral vein on the same side as the Watchman delivery sheath, so that hemostasis for both punctures can be achieved with a single figure-8 suture.

TRANSSEPTAL ACCESS AND PLACING INTRACARDIAC ECHOCARDIOGRAPHY IN THE LEFT ATRIUM

There are 2 main methods to obtain transseptal access for ICE placement in the LA. For both methods, the authors first place ICE in the RA and a long sheath SL1 (Abbott), or Preface (Biosense Webster) in the superior vena cava. ICE-guided transseptal access then is performed with a Baylis needle (Baylis Medical Mississauga, Ontario, Canada) or Brockenbrough 1 needle (Medtronic, Dublin, Ireland). When performing transseptal puncture with TEE, the bicaval view is used to assess the superior to inferior placement of the puncture while the short-axis view of the aortic valve is used to assess the anterior-posterior location. Although a low and posterior puncture often is recommended, in the authors' experience, if the puncture is too posterior, LAA cannulation can be more difficult. When using an ICE-guided approach, maximal tenting and puncture on an ICE view that shows the LAA or the ridge between the LAA and left pulmonary veins are aimed for, allowing a smooth trajectory toward the LAA. The authors avoid puncture posterior to the left pulmonary veins and aim to puncture low in the fossa.

After transseptal puncture, the sheath then is exchanged over a stiff wire (Amplatz Super Stiff, Boston Scientific, St. Paul, Minnesota) placed in the left superior pulmonary vein (LSPV) or over a ProTrak Pigtail wire (Baylis Medical), which forms a coil in the LA, for the Watchman sheath. The Watchman sheath then is used to dilate the septum. Septal dilatation is critical to allow advancement of the ICE catheter into the LA and may require several dilations. After adequate dilation, the Watchman sheath then is retracted back into the RA with the transseptal wire remaining in the LA. The ICE catheter then is advanced into the LA. This can be achieved under ICE guidance alone by deflecting (usually anterior flexion) the ICE tip toward the septum toward the image of the wire and with fluoroscopic guidance again using the wire as a guide. The Watchman sheath then is advanced again over the wire into the LA. Thus, both the Watchman sheath and ICE catheter pass through the same puncture.

The second approach to transseptal access involves making 2 separate transseptal punctures, both under ICE guidance. This approach requires 3 femoral venous punctures (1 for ICE and 2 for transseptal sheaths). An 8F AcuNav ICE catheter then can be placed into the LA via an 8.5F SL1 (Abbott, Chicago, Illinois) or a 9F or 10F ICE catheter can be placed through a 10F SL1. After the ICE catheter is in, the LA the sheath is pulled back to the septum or RA to allow maximum maneuverability of the catheter. The starting point of the ICE catheter is in the mid-LA. If a dual transseptal puncture method is used, too high a puncture for the sheath that accommodates the ICE catheter can make it more difficult to obtain the mitral annular ICE view, described later.

LEARNING HOW TO INCORPORATE INTRACARDIAC ECHOCARDIOGRAPHY FOR LEFT ATRIAL APPENDAGE CLOSURE

When first staring with an ICE-guided approach to LAAC placement, the authors suggest obtaining a preprocedure CT of the LA and appendage for an initial patient so that the operator can become familiarized with 3-D navigation of the ICE catheter in the LA. The authors initially did this in patients presenting for AF ablation in order to become experienced with catheter manipulation and obtaining proper views. With Biosense CARTO (Biosense Webster) patches placed on the patient and use of a SoundStar catheter (Biosense Webster), an ultrasound-guided map of the LA can be created after advancing the ICE catheter into the LA. This ultrasound map then can be merged with the CT. Then the ICE imaging plane can be superimposed on the CT (**Fig. 1**A, B), so the operator can better visualize how to manipulate the catheter.

INTRACARDIAC ECHOCARDIOGRAPHY–GUIDED VIEWS OF THE LEFT ATRIUM

Variable methods exist for imaging of the appendage during LAAC closure. Although there is some correlation between TEE and ICE views, the goal is not to replicate TEE views but instead to have adequate orthogonal ICE views to meet criteria for device release. In a registry of ICE-guided Amplatzer Amulet implantation, device imaging was highly variable and occurred from either the right atrium (RA), LA, LSPV, and pulmonary artery, depending on operator preference.[14] Although ICE-guided implantation solely from the RA has been described with high success rates (>97.5%) with skilled operators,[24,25] it often does not provide sufficient visualization of the depth and width of the appendage, especially in patients with LA enlargement or a thick fossa ovalis. In addition, it is inadequate to assess for appendage thrombus. Imaging from the pulmonary artery provides excellent views of the appendage given its anatomic proximity but must be approached cautiously as to avoid perforation.[26] Placement of ICE in the coronary sinus[27] offers a limited imaging plane due to movement constraints and a long-axis view is difficult to obtain. For this reason and for the risk of perforation, the authors avoid ICE placement in the coronary sinus.

Different LA ICE views have been described for LAAC. Alkhouli and colleagues[12] describe a simplified 2-view method from the LA, which provides a long-axis view with the ICE catheter in the mid-LA (analogous to 45°–90° TEE view) and a short-axis view from the mitral valve, which is analogous to the 135° TEE view. Device release was based successfully on only these 2 views, and this method removes the need for advancement of the ICE catheter into the pulmonary vein, which the investigators argue may confer a safety benefit and may be less technically challenging for less advanced ICE users.

The Watchman FLX was FDA approved in 2020. Among multiple design enhancements, including full recapture and repositioning, it has a ball-like shape that can be advanced and allows more proximal device placement. Korsholm and colleagues[28] describe ICE-guided implantation of Watchman FLX using a 3-view approach. They used the mid-LA long-axis view, a view from the catheter in the LSPV, and a supramitral view. Device release criteria were determined by at least 2 views, 1 of which was from the supramitral position. With the combination of preprocedural CT, ICE-guided implantation, and the enhanced design of the Watchman FLX device, first device implant success was 96%. This study demonstrates that although advances in ICE imaging would be welcome to facilitate LAAC, enhancements of the device itself and device delivery allow high first implant success rates with current imaging quality. The authors' preferred approach is to use 3 views from the LA, including a mid-LA long-axis home view, a

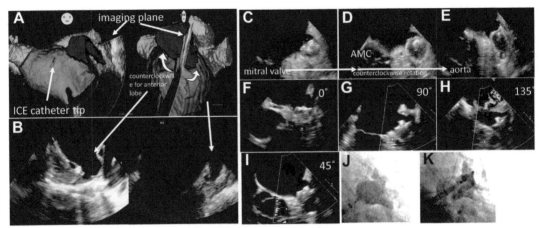

Fig. 1. Home ICE view of the LAA. (*A*) Home LA view, shown in a 3-D rendition of the LA. The ICE catheter tip is positioned in the mid-LA, with the imaging plane facing toward the LAA (*left*). In a left anterior oblique view (*right*), the imaging plane cuts through the LAA. Clockwise rotation directs the imaging plane toward the posterior lobe, whereas counterclockwise rotation would show the anterior lobe. The tip of the LA ridge is visible. (*B*) corresponding ICE images. (*C–E*) Watchman deployment from the home view. Serial images in a different patient obtained by gradual counterclockwise rotation from the posterior lobe-mitral valve view (*C*), showing the aortomitral continuity, and the aortic valve, with the LAA and Watchman in different angles. (*F–I*) TEE views obtained at 45 days postimplant. (*J*, *K*) LAA angiograms before and after Watchman deployment in a right anterior oblique caudal view.

view from the LSPV,[29] and third supramitral view with the ICE imaging plane facing upward toward the appendage.

VIEW 1: HOME VIEW

The first view obtained with ICE is referred to as the home view (see **Fig. 1**). This view is related most closely to the 45° to 90° view on TEE with the plane of imaging cutting through the mitral valve and LAA (**Table 2**). The ICE catheter tip initially is placed in the middle of the LA body. It then is rotated until the mitral annulus and appendage come into view. A slight rightward and/or posterior tilt may be needed to fully bring the appendage into. From this view, initial measurements are made of the LAA ostial diameter. Measurements are made from the left circumflex or mitral valve annulus to a point that is 2 cm below the tip of the ridge. The lobes can be brought into view by rotating the catheter clockwise or counterclockwise, respectively, as shown in **Fig. 1**A, B. Counterclockwise rotation shows the anterior LAA lobe, adjacent to the aorta, whereas clockwise rotation shows the posterior LAA lobe, commonly over the basal left ventricle (LV), and frequently visualizing the mitral valve and the blood vessels at the LV base–circumflex coronary artery and the great cardiac vein. It is important to scan across the appendage in this manner to fully appreciate the anatomy and depth of the appendage.

The LA home view provides some images that closely correlate with those obtained by TEE. **Fig. 1** shows a series of images obtained from the LA view. Starting from a posterior orientation imaging the mitral valve and posterior lobe of the LAA, the Watchman position can be visualized (see **Fig. 1**C). By rotating the ICE probe counterclockwise, successive views of the Watchman are obtained until it can be seen adjacent to the aortic valve (see **Fig. 1**E). A TEE obtained 45 days postimplant demonstrates a close match between the 90° view on TEE (see **Fig. 1**G) and the posterior lobe view by ICE (see **Fig. 1**C). Similarly, the 45° view on TEE (see **Fig. 1**I) closely matches the image of the anterior LAA lobe after counterclockwise rotation (see **Fig. 1**E).

VIEW 2: LEFT SUPERIOR PULMONARY VEIN VIEW

The LA home view may be inadequate to visualize the depth of the LAA, or it may not be stable enough. For this purpose, the authors insert the ICE catheter in the LSPV, which in most cases runs parallel and in close proximity to the LAA. To do so, from the home view, the authors rotate the ICE catheter clockwise until the pulmonary veins are visualized, using the carina as an easily identifiable landmark. Then the catheter is advanced into the LSPV and rotated counterclockwise to face anteriorly toward the LAA. Note that

Table 2
Relation between intracardiac echocardiography, transesophageal echocardiography, and fluoroscopy views

Intracardiac Echocardiography View	Approximate Transesophageal Echocardiography View	Approximate Fluoroscopy View	Maneuver
View 1: LA home view, long-axis LAA	45°-90°	Right anterior oblique 30° ± cranial angulation	Place ICE in mid-LA, rotate to see mitral valve and LAA
View 2: LSPV view	0°-90°	Right anterior oblique 30° ± cranial angulation	Clockwise from home view until see ridge between LAA and LSPV and then slowly advance ICE catheter into LSPV. Once in LSPV counterclockwise, and initially see posterior lobe and then anterior lobe with continued counterclockwise torque
View 3: mitral annular view	135°	Right anterior oblique 20° Caudal 20°	From home view, deflect ICE catheter down toward mitral valve and advance toward mitral valve. Then relax deflection, and rotate imaging plane upward (counterclockwise) to face appendage.

the trajectory of the ICE catheter from the inferior vena cava, through the septum and into the LSPV, would constrain the catheter shaft at an angle similar to the 45° TEE view. Although the ultrasound beam is facing anteriorly, deflecting the catheter rightward would then flatten it out matching the 0° view on TEE, whereas deflecting it leftward would make it approach 90°. Still, most of the imaging is performed as was for the home view, by rotating the catheter counterclockwise or clockwise. **Fig. 2** shows examples of LSPV views. With a clockwise turn, the posterior LAA lobe is visualized, next to the mitral valve (see **Fig. 2C**). Counterclockwise rotation shows the deeper anterior lobe, which enables insertion of the sheath over the pigtail catheter (see **Fig. 2D**). Upon Watchman deployment, device location, seal (with Doppler) and compression can be assessed (see **Fig. 2F–H**). The ICE catheter also can be advanced into the left inferior pulmonary vein, with subsequent manipulation similar to that used from the LSPV.[11] Imaging, however, tends to be limited to the posterior LAA lobe and not always is stable.

Between the home view and the LSPV view, the authors chose the view with the best imaging and most stable position to serve as the working view for the procedure.

VIEW 3: 135° OR INTRACARDIAC ECHOCARDIOGRAPHY ON MITRAL VALVE VIEW

The third view places the ICE catheter across the mitral valve in the basal LV, with the imaging plane facing superiorly at the LAA from below (**Fig. 3**). From the LA home view, the mitral valve view is obtained by deflecting the ICE catheter down and rotating it counterclockwise while advancing the catheter tip into the LV. The authors have found it easiest to use the ICE catheters own images to guide this maneuver, by visualizing the mitral valve en face, deflecting the catheter toward it (usually anterior torque) and advancing. In this manner, the LV is entered easily, but the imaging plane faces downward toward the LV inferior wall upon entry. To image the LAA, the catheter deflection is relaxed and the shaft is rotated until the LAA comes into the image. In this view, the closest structures visualized are the LV base, the circumflex artery, and great cardiac vein, with the LAA below (see **Fig. 3C**). Counterclockwise rotation

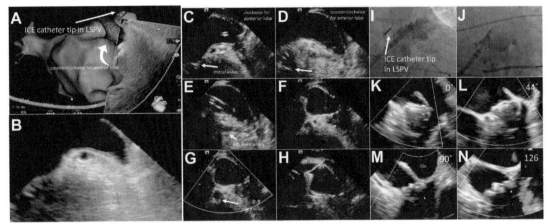

Fig. 2. View of LAA from LSPV. (*A*) The imaging plane faces the LAA from the LSPV, and counterclockwise rotation brings the anterior lobe into plane. (*B*) Corresponding ICE image. Watchman deployment from LSPV (*C–N*). (*C*). Initial view from LSPV in a different patient. Note the LA ridge is seen closest to the transducer and the ridge tip is not visible. The mitral valve is seen next to the LAA posterior lobe with a portion of the pigtail catheter. (*D*) Anterior LAA lobe shown after counterclockwise rotation. The full LAA depth is appreciated, and sheath insertion follows. (*E*) Note the aortic root and proximity to the left main coronary artery. (*F–H*). Watchman deployment follows (*F*), and its position can be verified by clockwise rotation toward the posterior lobe (*G*) with Doppler interrogation for leaks, and final release (*H*). (*I, J*). LAA angiography showing ICE catheter location and after deployment. (*K–N*). TEE images 45 days postdeployment showing optimal device position and seal.

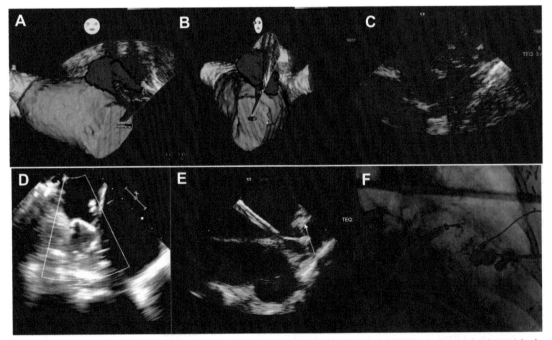

Fig. 3. View 3, or mitral annular view. (*A*) The tip of the ICE catheter is in LV just beyond mitral valve with the imaging plane facing toward the appendage in AP (*A*) and left lateral (*B*). (*C*) ICE image from (*A*) and (*B*) . (*D*) TEE 135° view from a different patient. (*E*) Mitral annular ICE view of deployed Watchman allowing accurate ostial measurement. (*F*) Right anterior oblique caudal fluoroscopic view, which is most related to 135° TEE view and mitral annular ICE view.

would show the posterior LAA lobe, whereas clockwise rotation can bring the anterior lobe into the image. This view can resemble the 135° view on TEE (see **Fig. 3**D). In the authors' experience, however, the catheter position often is unstable in this view and it is not suited to serve as a working view for the majority of the procedure but rather as a confirmatory view of position (see **Fig. 3**E), seal, and compression.

Although the home view and LSPV view offer similar imaging planes, the mitral valve view is critical to obtain because it offers complementary imaging to the prior views and mimics the high-angle 135 TEE view, which is helpful in visualizing a mitral shoulder. High-angle views are particularly important for the Watchman FLX because a significant shoulder is discouraged to avoid insufficient radial force on the device. If the mitral valve view cannot be obtained, then a right anterior oblique caudal image with contrast angiography can be used to ascertain the needed information.

USE OF FLUOROSCOPY DURING THE PROCEDURE

The fluoroscopy corelates with TEE are as follows: the 0° view is similar to an anterior posterior cranial view, the 45° view is similar to a right anterior oblique cranial view, the 90° view is similar to a right anterior oblique view, and the 135° view is similar to a right anterior oblique caudal view. The authors integrate ICE views with fluoroscopy to fully appreciate appendage anatomy (see **Table 2**). The right anterior oblique caudal view often serves as the working view for the procedure. This view is most related to the mitral annular ICE view. The home view and LSPV views are most related

fluoroscopically to right anterior oblique with or without cranial angulation.

THE DIFFICULT APPENDAGE

Arguably, one of the most difficult LAA anatomies to occlude with Watchman is one in which a short LAA neck is followed by a lobe running posterior to the pulmonary artery. The difficulty arises from the complex imaging interpretation and the fact that, despite usually sufficient LAA depth, the lobe orientation is nearly parallel to the LA roof and, therefore, not a useable depth because the sheath cannot be inserted in it. Additionally, the proximal LAA neck opens sideways to the retro-pulmonary artery lobe, and, when the Watchman is deployed too distally, it can expand into the lobe without any compression. **Fig. 4** shows an example.

ADVANCES IN INTRACARDIAC ECHOCARDIOGRAPHY IMAGING

The 3-D ICE probes are under development and have the advantage of multiplanar imaging without having to alter the ICE catheter position. The 3-D ICE catheter ACUSON AcuNav (Siemens, Chicago, IL) is 12F. It can be placed directly across the transseptal access site into the LA or via a 14F sheath (Cook, Bloomington, IN). Either way it requires a larger transseptal puncture. After a limited market release, its development was discontinued by the manufacturer. A novel 4-dimensional ICE catheter, NuVision (NuVera medical, Los Gatos, California), recently has been developed. The catheter allows real time 3-D imaging of LA structures with a 90° × 90° field of view.

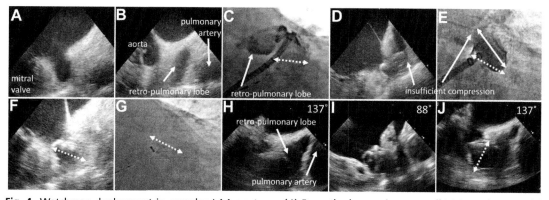

Fig. 4. Watchman deployment in complex LAA anatomy. (*A*) From the home view, a small LAA can be seen. (*B*) Ccounterclockwise rotation shows an LAA lobe between aorta and pulmonary artery, confirmed by LAA angiography (*C*). LAA neck (*dotted line*) marks desired Watchman deployment. (*D, E*) Initial deployment is too deep and the Watchman expands in the lobe, distal to the LAA neck, with insufficient compression. (*F, G*) After recapture and redeployment, adequate position and compression are shown. (*H–J*) TEE images before (*H*) and 45 days after, showing optimal device position.

The utility of 3-D ICE for LAAC still is to be determined, but it allows an en face view of the LAA ostium from the LA, which can be used to measure diameters in long axis and short axis at once.

SUMMARY

Although TEE was the original imaging modality during trials of LAAC, its use requires more coordination and adds more complexity to the procedure. ICE offers sufficient orthogonal views to accurately assess LAAC and is a familiar tool for most electrophysiologists. Multiple studies have shown the safety and efficacy of ICE-guided closure. In addition, it creates procedural efficiencies and is cost effective. As LAAC procedures become increasing common, ICE-based imaging will be an invaluable skill to facilitate appendage closure.

REFERENCES

1. Reddy VY, Doshi SK, Sievert H, et al. Percutaneous left atrial appendage closure for stroke prophylaxis in patients with atrial fibrillation: 2.3-year follow-up of the PROTECT AF (watchman left atrial appendage system for embolic protection in patients with atrial fibrillation) trial. Circulation 2013;127(6):720–9.
2. Holmes DR Jr, Kar S, Price MJ, et al. Prospective randomized evaluation of the Watchman Left Atrial Appendage Closure device in patients with atrial fibrillation versus long-term warfarin therapy: the PREVAIL trial. J Am Coll Cardiol 2014;64(1):1–12.
3. Reddy VY, Doshi SK, Kar S, et al. 5-Year outcomes after left atrial appendage closure: from the PREVAIL and PROTECT AF trials. J Am Coll Cardiol 2017;70(24):2964–75.
4. Reddy VY, Gibson DN, Kar S, et al. Post-approval U.S. Experience with left atrial appendage closure for stroke prevention in atrial fibrillation. J Am Coll Cardiol 2017;69(3):253–61.
5. De Caterina R, Husted S, Wallentin L, et al. New oral anticoagulants in atrial fibrillation and acute coronary syndromes: ESC Working Group on Thrombosis-Task Force on Anticoagulants in Heart Disease position paper. J Am Coll Cardiol 2012; 59(16):1413–25.
6. Ruff CT, Giugliano RP, Braunwald E, et al. Comparison of the efficacy and safety of new oral anticoagulants with warfarin in patients with atrial fibrillation: a meta-analysis of randomised trials. Lancet 2014; 383(9921):955–62.
7. Osmancik P, Herman D, Neuzil P, et al. Left atrial appendage closure versus direct oral anticoagulants in high-risk patients with atrial fibrillation. J Am Coll Cardiol 2020;75(25):3122–35.
8. Hildick-Smith D, Landmesser U, Camm AJ, et al. Left atrial appendage occlusion with the Amplatzer™ Amulet™ device: full results of the prospective global observational study. Eur Heart J 2020;41(30):2894–901.
9. January CT, Wann LS, Calkins H, et al. 2019 AHA/ ACC/HRS focused update of the 2014 AHA/ACC/ HRS Guideline for the Management of patients with atrial fibrillation: a report of the American College of Cardiology/American Heart Association Task Force on Clinical Practice Guidelines and the Heart Rhythm Society. J Am Coll Cardiol 2019; 74(1):104–32.
10. Benjamin EJ, Muntner P, Alonso A, et al. Heart disease and stroke statistics-2019 update: a report from the American Heart Association. Circulation 2019;139(10):e56–528.
11. Hemam ME, Kuroki K, Schurmann PA, et al. Left atrial appendage closure with the Watchman device using intracardiac vs transesophageal echocardiography: procedural and cost considerations. Heart Rhythm 2019;16(3):334–42.
12. Alkhouli M, Chaker Z, Alqahtani F, et al. Outcomes of Routine intracardiac echocardiography to guide left atrial appendage occlusion. JACC Clin Electrophysiol 2020;6(4):393–400.
13. Frangieh AH, Alibegovic J, Templin C, et al. Intracardiac versus transesophageal echocardiography for left atrial appendage occlusion with watchman. Catheter Cardiovasc Interv 2017;90(2):331–8.
14. Berti S, Pastormerlo LE, Santoro G, et al. Intracardiac versus transesophageal echocardiographic guidance for left atrial appendage occlusion: the LAAO Italian multicenter registry. JACC Cardiovasc Interv 2018;11(11):1086–92.
15. Velagapudi P, Turagam MK, Kolte D, et al. Intracardiac vs transesophageal echocardiography for percutaneous left atrial appendage occlusion: a meta-analysis. J Cardiovasc Electrophysiol 2019; 30(4):461–7.
16. Matsuo Y, Neuzil P, Petru J, et al. Left atrial appendage closure under intracardiac echocardiographic guidance: feasibility and comparison with transesophageal echocardiography. J Am Heart Assoc 2016;5(10):e003695.
17. Mosleh W, Sheikh A, Said Z, et al. The use of cardiac-CT alone to exclude left atrial thrombus before atrial fibrillation ablation: efficiency, safety, and cost analysis. Pacing Clin Electrophysiol 2018; 41(7):727–33.
18. Romero J, Husain SA, Kelesidis I, et al. Detection of left atrial appendage thrombus by cardiac computed tomography in patients with atrial fibrillation: a meta-analysis. Circ Cardiovasc Imaging 2013;6(2):185–94.
19. Patel A, Au E, Donegan K, et al. Multidetector row computed tomography for identification of left atrial

appendage filling defects in patients undergoing pulmonary vein isolation for treatment of atrial fibrillation: comparison with transesophageal echocardiography. Heart Rhythm 2008;5(2):253–60.

20. Gilhofer TS, Saw J. Periprocedural imaging for left atrial appendage closure: computed tomography, transesophageal echocardiography, and intracardiac echocardiography. Card Electrophysiol Clin 2020;12(1):55–65.

21. Eng MH, Wang DD, Greenbaum AB, et al. Prospective, randomized comparison of 3-dimensional computed tomography guidance versus TEE data for left atrial appendage occlusion (PRO3DLAAO). Catheter Cardiovasc Interv 2018;92(2):401–7.

22. Baran J, Stec S, Pilichowska-Paszkiet E, et al. Intracardiac echocardiography for detection of thrombus in the left atrial appendage: comparison with transesophageal echocardiography in patients undergoing ablation for atrial fibrillation: the Action-Ice I Study. Circ Arrhythm Electrophysiol 2013;6(6):1074–81.

23. Anter E, Silverstein J, Tschabrunn CM, et al. Comparison of intracardiac echocardiography and transesophageal echocardiography for imaging of the right and left atrial appendages. Heart Rhythm 2014;11(11):1890–7.

24. Berti S, Paradossi U, Meucci F, et al. Periprocedural intracardiac echocardiography for left atrial appendage closure: a dual-center experience. JACC Cardiovasc Interv 2014;7(9):1036–44.

25. Prakash R, Saw J. Imaging for percutaneous left atrial appendage closure. Catheter Cardiovasc Interv 2018;92(2):437–50.

26. MacDonald ST, Newton JD, Ormerod OJ. Intracardiac echocardiography off piste? Closure of the left atrial appendage using ICE and local anesthesia. Catheter Cardiovasc Interv 2011;77(1): 124–7.

27. Melman YF, Foppa M, Huang H, et al. Visualization of the left atrial appendage from the coronary sinus by intracardiac echocardiography. Heart Rhythm 2014;11(9):1603–4.

28. Korsholm K, Samaras A, Andersen A, et al. The Watchman FLX Device: First European Experience and Feasibility of Intracardiac Echocardiography to Guide Implantation. JACC Clin Electrophysiol 2020 Dec 14;6(13):1633–42.

29. Patti G, Mantione L, Goffredo C, et al. Intracardiac echocardiography with ultrasound probe placed in the upper left pulmonary vein to guide left atrial appendage closure: first description. Catheter Cardiovasc Interv 2019;93(1):169–73.

Intracardiac Echocardiography to Guide Catheter Ablation of Idiopathic Ventricular Arrythmias

Matthew Hanson, MD, Andres Enriquez, MD*

KEYWORDS

- Intracardiac echocardiography • Catheter ablation • Idiopathic ventricular arrythmias

KEY POINTS

- The RVOT is the most common source of ventricular arrhythmias in patients without structural heart disease and the site of origin often lies above the pulmonary valve. ICE is helpful to determine the location of the ablation catheter relative to the valve plane and proximity to the left coronary artery.
- When ablating the LV ostium, especially the aortic cusp region, ICE allows to delineate the origin and proximal course of the coronary arteries, minimizing the risk of coronary artery injury and often obviating the need for coronary angiography.
- LV summit and para-Hisian VAs often need to be targeted from neighboring structures. In these cases, ICE provides a good understanding of the anatomical relationship between adjacent structures.
- ICE has a particularly key role for ablation of intracavitary structures such as the moderator band and RV/LV papillary muscles, ensuring adequate contact with the structure of interest and monitoring catheter stability during the cardiac cycle.

INTRODUCTION

Catheter ablation has become a first-line therapy for idiopathic ventricular arrhythmias (VAs),[1] and a thorough understanding of the anatomic substrate is key for a safe and successful procedure.

Intracardiac echocardiography (ICE) allows real-time visualization of cardiac structures and provides an accurate assessment of anatomic relationships, which may be complex and not always intuitive.[2] The understanding of these relationships allows more targeted mapping, minimizes the risk of collateral damage, and provides the opportunity to ablate certain arrhythmias from neighboring structures. ICE is also valuable for ensuring adequate catheter-tissue contact during ablation, monitoring lesion formation, and, in combination with electroanatomic mapping, has the potential to reduce or eliminate the need for fluoroscopy.

This article describes the application of ICE as part of an anatomy-guided approach to mapping and ablating idiopathic ventricular tachycardia (VT) and premature ventricular complexes (PVCs).

RIGHT VENTRICULAR OUTFLOW TRACT AND PULMONARY ARTERY

The right ventricular outflow tract (RVOT) or right ventricular (RV) infundibulum is the most common site of origin of idiopathic VAs, accounting for 70% to 80% of all cases.[3] In recent years, it has been suggested that a significant proportion of these arrhythmias actually originate above the pulmonary valve (PV) level, from myocardial sleeves extending into the pulmonary cusps.[4,5]

Anatomically, the RVOT is a tubular structure located anterior and leftward relative to the left ventricular outflow tract (LVOT).[6,7] It is composed

Division of Cardiology, Queen's University, Kingston, Ontario, Canada
* Corresponding author. Division of Cardiology, Queen's University, 76 Stuart Street, Kingston, Ontario K7L 2V7, Canada.
E-mail address: Andres.Enriquez@kingstonhsc.ca

Card Electrophysiol Clin 13 (2021) 325–335
https://doi.org/10.1016/j.ccep.2021.03.010

of a free wall (anterior) and a septal wall (posterior), which wraps around the aortic root. The inferior and most rightward portion is continuous with the tricuspid annulus and the interventricular septum, where the bundle of His is located. Its most superior and leftward portion is adjacent to the left coronary cusp (LCC), in close proximity to the left anterior descending (LAD) and anterior interventricular vein (AIV).

The PV is superior and leftward of the aortic valve (AoV) and consists of 3 cusps: anterior (APC), right (RPC), and left (LPC).[6] The RPC lies at variable distance from, and is sometimes adjacent to, the right atrial appendage. The APC is the most superficial and lies immediately beneath the pericardium, with no other cardiac structures related to it. The LPC has the most important anatomic relationships; it is in close proximity to the left main coronary artery (LMCA) on the epicardial surface of the left ventricle (LV) and the left atrial (LA) appendage. This relationship explains why some LV summit arrhythmias can be eliminated by ablation within the LPC.[8] For the same reason, coronary angiography is often recommended when ablating above the valve level.

When imaging the outflow tracts region, it should be noted that the PV is oriented on a perpendicular plane with respect to the AoV; therefore, when the AoV is displayed in short-axis, the PV is seen on long-axis, and vice versa. In addition, the PV lies on an oblique transverse plane, with the LPC being more inferior than the other 2 cusps.

The following ICE views are useful to guide ablation of RVOT and pulmonary artery (PA) arrhythmias[2,9]:

a. Home view: It is obtained with the ICE catheter in the midright atrium (RA) in the neutral position and the transducer oriented anteriorly (**Fig. 1**A). It provides an image of the RA, tricuspid valve (TV), aortic root, and the RV inflow and outflow tracts. The 2 aortic cusps visualized in this view are the noncoronary cusp (NCC) and right coronary cusp (RCC).

b. Short-axis view of the PV: It is obtained by advancing the ICE catheter 1 to 2 cm from the home view while applying some clockwise rotation and rightward tilt (**Fig. 1**B). This maneuver positions the catheter tip at the level of the RA appendage. In this view, the cusp that is closest to the aortic root is the LPC; the farthest from the aorta is the APC, and the cusp oriented to the right side (away from the LV) is the RPC. The AoV is displayed in the long-axis and the 2 cusps visualized in this plane are the NCC and LCC. We also call this view the "summit view,"

as it is very helpful to ablate LV summit arrhythmias (see later discussion).

c. Long-axis view of the PV: It is the best projection to determine the location of the ablation catheter respect to the PV. This view is obtained by advancing the ICE catheter across the TV into the RV, followed by clockwise rotation. The first 2 pulmonary cusps to be visualized are the LPC (adjacent to the aortic root) and the APC (also called nonseptal), which are the 2 more leftward of the 3 cusps (**Fig. 1**C). The RPC can be seen in isolation with further rotation (**Fig. 1**D).

VAs from the RVOT and PA can be targeted using a direct approach (**Fig. 2**) or a "reversed U-curve" technique, which is particularly useful when the site of origin lies above the valve level (**Fig. 3**). In this technique, the ablation catheter is advanced into the PA and then deflected in a "candy cane" shape using the D-curve,[10] thus providing better contact and stability, minimizing also the risk of coronary artery injury.

LEFT VENTRICULAR OSTIUM

Basal LV structures are part of the LV ostium, a term coined by McAlpine[11] to describe the elliptical opening that forms the base of the LV. It is covered by the aortoventricular membrane, a tough fibrous structure that is perforated by the aorta anteriorly and the mitral valve (MV) posterior and laterally. The AoV occupies a central location within the heart and is composed of 3 cusps.[6] From an attitudinal perspective, the RCC is the most anterior and inferior cusp relative to the sternum; the NCC is posterior and rightward, and the LCC is posterior and leftward. The RCC is in close proximity to the posteroseptal aspect of the RVOT, whereas the LCC is adjacent to the anterior aspect of the LV ostium, close to the LAD and the AIV/great cardiac vein junction from the epicardial surface. On the other side, the NCC is in relationship with both the left and the right atria separated by the interatrial septum. Below the commissure between the RCC and NCC lies the membranous ventricular septum, where the penetrating bundle of His is located.

In contrast to the RVOT, which is comprised entirely of muscle, the ventriculoaortic junction is composed of a fibrous portion and a muscular portion.[12,13] The muscular portion, more extensive, corresponds to the interventricular muscular septum and is under the RCC and the anterior half of the LCC. The fibrous portion corresponds to the aortomitral continuity (AMC), a curtain of fibrous tissue that extends between the anterior

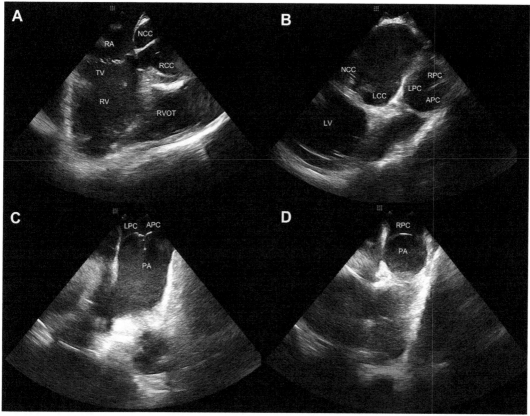

Fig. 1. ICE visualization of the RVOT and PA. (*A*) Home view. (*B*) Short-axis view of the PV. (*C,D*) Long-axis view of the PV.

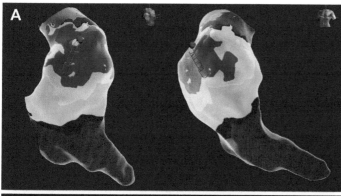

Fig. 2. Example of PVC ablated from the RVOT free wall, below the APC. (*A*) Activation map of the PVC showing site of successful ablation. (*B*) ICE images demonstrate the position of the catheter below the valvular plane, in relation to the APC. AO, aorta; RPA, right pulmonary artery.

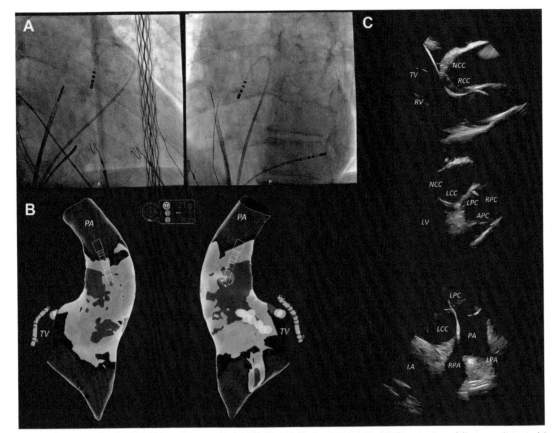

Fig. 3. Example of VT ablation from the LPC. (*A*). Right anterior oblique and left anterior oblique radiographic views of the ablation catheter at the successful ablation site using a "reversed U-curve" approach. (*B*) Activation map showing earliest site of activation; His cloud is marked with yellow dots. (*C*) Catheter position in different ICE views (from top to bottom: home view, PV short-axis, and PV long-axis). LPA, left pulmonary artery.

leaflet of the MV and the noncoronary and LCCs of the AoV. VAs may originate from the muscle of the LV ostium, and they can be mapped and/or ablated directly from the subvalvular LV endocardium or indirectly from the coronary cusps or the coronary venous circulation.

LV ostial structures can be imaged by advancing the ICE catheter into the RV, followed by deflection release and clockwise rotation of the handpiece (**Figs. 4–6**). The following views will be obtained in sequence:

a. MV view (see **Fig. 4**A): This view shows part of the LA, both MV leaflets and often the anterolateral papillary muscle (ALPM), an oblique view of the LVOT, and the adjacent RVOT separated by the infundibular septum.
b. Subannular LVOT and AMC (see **Fig. 4**B): Additional clockwise rotation produces a short-axis view of the LVOT at the subvalvular plane level. The interface between the mitral and aortic annuli corresponds to the AMC.

c. Annular LVOT and short-axis view of the AoV (see **Fig. 4**C): It is the best view to guide ablation of aortic cusp VAs. In this view, the cusp that is closest on the image to the transducer is the RCC, which is adjacent to the RVOT. The cusp that is farthest from the transducer is the LCC, which is in close proximity to the LA appendage, and the NCC is adjacent to the LA. The junction between the RCC and LCC is surrounded by a portion of myocardial tissue that is part of the LV ostium and is the most common source of LVOT arrhythmias.[14] From this view, additional clockwise rotation produces a long-axis view of the aortic root, which allows localization of the ablation catheter relative to the valve plane and is helpful when advancing the catheter into the LV cavity.

LEFT VENTRICULAR SUMMIT

The LV summit, as described by McAlpine, is the highest portion of the LV epicardium, above the

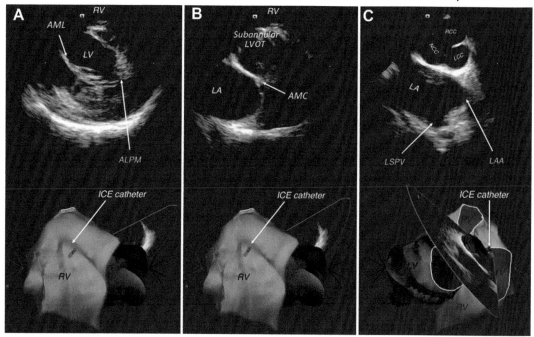

Fig. 4. ICE imaging of basal left ventricular structures with corresponding CARTOSOUND (Biosense-Webster, Diamond Bar, CA, USA) maps. (*A*) MV view. (*B*) Subannular LVOT and AMC. (*C*) Annular LVOT and short-axis view of the AoV. ALPM, anterolateral papillary muscle; AML, anterior mitral leaflet; LAA, left atria appendage; LSPV, left superior pulmonary vein.

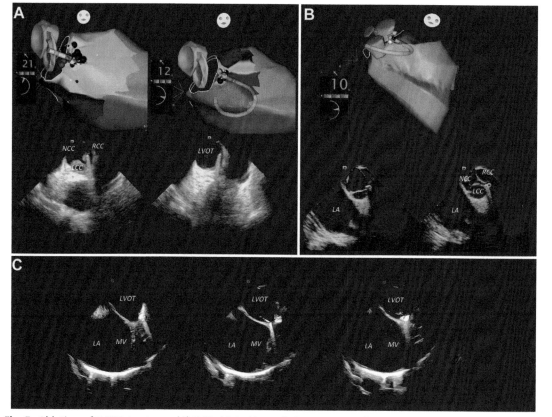

Fig. 5. Ablation of LVOT structures. (*A*) PVC ablated by radiofrequency application at the RCC, above (*left panel*) and below the valve plane (*right panel*). (*B*) Successful ablation of PVC from the right-left cusp commissure. (*C*) PVC ablated at the AMC; note lesion formation after the initial radiofrequency application.

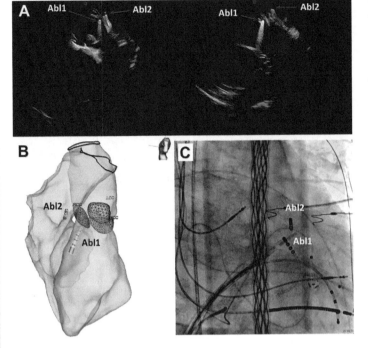

Fig. 6. Use of ICE to guide bipolar ablation of intramural periaortic VT. (*A*) ICE showing the position of the 2 ablation catheters at the subaortic LVOT, immediately below the RCC (Abl1), and the septal RVOT, below the LPC (Abl2). (*B, C*) Electroanatomic map and right anterior oblique radiographic view showing the relationship between the catheters.

upper end of the anterior interventricular sulcus and bounded by the bifurcation between the LAD and left circumflex artery (LCX). It is a common site of origin of idiopathic VAs, and despite its epicardial location, catheter ablation from the epicardium is rarely successful because of proximity to the coronary arteries and the presence of thick epicardial fat. Therefore, in most cases, LV summit arrhythmias must be targeted from the coronary venous system or adjacent endocardial structures, such as the LCC, the subaortic LV, or the LPC. As previously mentioned, "the summit view" is obtained by slightly advancing the ICE catheter from the home view, followed by clockwise rotation and also some rightward tilt (**Fig. 7**). This view provides adequate visualization of these endocardial neighbors and may be helpful if simultaneous unipolar ablation or bipolar ablation from 2 different structures is considered.

Coronary artery injury is a rare but serious complication of ablation in the outflow tracts.[15] The LMCA or proximal LAD can be damaged by ablation in the LCC, PA, or LV summit (epicardially or via the distal coronary venous system), while the right coronary artery (RCA) can be damaged by ablation in the RCC. ICE can provide an accurate assessment of the coronary anatomy, minimizing the risk of coronary artery injury and in many cases obviating coronary angiogram (**Fig. 8**). The ostium of the LMCA can be identified in the annular LVOT

view, typically at the same level that the LPC and APC are visualized. The course of its trunk and bifurcation into LAD and LCX can be followed by slight counterclockwise torque of the catheter. The RCA ostium can be visualized with the ICE catheter in the basal RV, applying some clockwise rotation from the aorta long-axis view or from the RA with some anterior and lateral torque.

PARA-HISIAN REGION AND POSTERIOR SUPERIOR PROCESS OF THE LEFT VENTRICLE

From an electrophysiology perspective, the para-Hisian region can be defined as the portion of the interventricular septum within 10 mm of the largest His bundle potential recording site.[16] The septal aspect of the tricuspid annulus and para-Hisian region can be imaged from the home view, sometimes with slight anterior angulation and clockwise torque of the ICE catheter (**Fig. 9**A). A long-axis view of the aortic root is obtained, where the cusp closest to the transducer is the NCC and the opposite cusp is the RCC. The 2 TV leaflets visualized in this view are the septal and posterior leaflets. The His region is immediately below the RCC-NCC junction, underneath the septal leaflet of the TV. Similar to LV summit arrhythmias, para-Hisian VAs often can be targeted from neighboring structures, which in this case include the RCC or NCC, the slow pathway region in the RA,

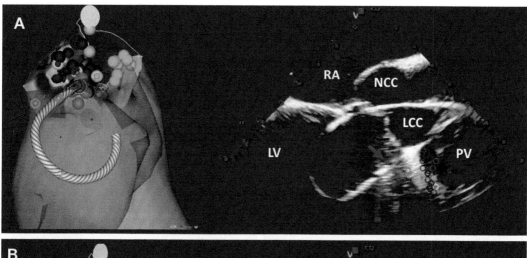

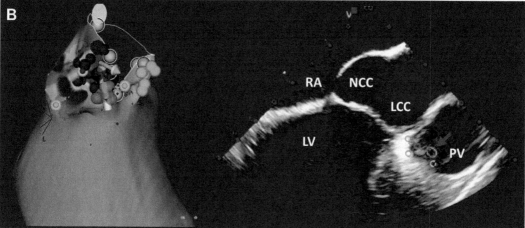

Fig. 7. Ablation of LV summit PVC by sequential radiofrequency application from the subaortic LV, immediately below the LCC (*A*), and from the RVOT, above and below the LPC (*B*). The tip of the ablation catheter is marked with an arrowhead. (Image courtesy Dr. Luis Saenz.)

the RV below the septal TV leaflet, or the basal septal LV. ICE provides a good understanding of the relationship between these structures.

Additional clockwise rotation from the home view will bring into view the interventricular septum and then the posterior superior process (PSP) of the LV, also referred to as basal inferoseptal LV process, which is the portion of the LV adjacent to the inferior and septal aspect of the RA.[17] The structures visualized in the "PSP view" include the RA, LV cavity, NCC, and LCC (**Fig. 10**). This anatomic relationship is relevant, as some VAs from this region may be ablated from the RA. In addition, it has been reported as a potential site for percutaneous LV access in patients with mechanical aortic and mitral prosthetic valves.[18]

TRICUSPID ANNULUS

The TV lies inferiorly and anteriorly to the MV and is composed of 3 leaflets: anterior (the largest),

posterior (the smallest), and septal. When described relative to their anatomic position in the body (attitudinally appropriate nomenclature), the 3 leaflets would be anterior-superior, inferior, and septal.[19]

The home view is the starting point to guide ablation of VAs from the tricuspid annulus. Slight clockwise rotation of the ICE catheter allows visualization of more septal aspect of the TV (simultaneous visualization of the TV and aortic root), while counterclockwise rotation brings into view the lateral annulus. An important role of ICE in this group of VAs is to assess the relationship between the ablation catheter and the valve leaflets, which may prevent adequate contact between the catheter tip and the subvalvular plane.

Ablation is particularly challenging at the superior and lateral regions of the TV and, in the authors' experience, a "reversed S-curve" technique is preferred in these cases (**Fig. 9**B).[20] In this technique, the ablation catheter is introduced through

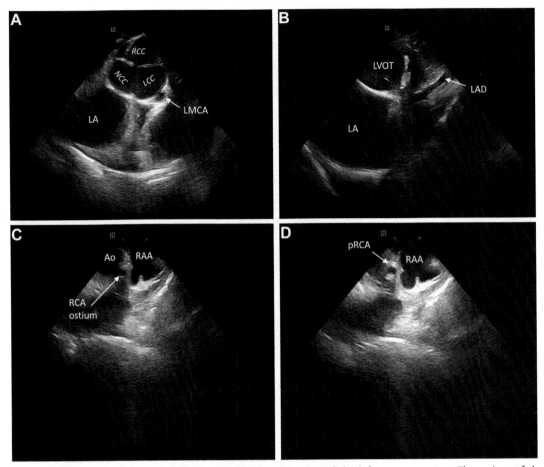

Fig. 8. ICE visualization of the coronary arteries. (*A,B*) Delineation of the left coronary artery. The ostium of the LMCA is visualized with the ICE catheter positioned at the base of the RVOT and the beam facing upwards to produce a short-axis view of the aortic valve. Slight counterclockwise rotation allows to follow the LMCA until its bifurcation into LAD and LCX. (*C,D*) Right coronary artery. The ostium of the RCA can be identified by applying gentle clockwise rotation from the aorta long-axis view. Additional clockwise rotation allows to follow the proximal course of the RCA as it approaches the AV groove. pRCA, proximal right coronary artery; RAA, right atrial appendage.

a deflectable sheath (usually an Agilis sheath, Abbott, St Paul, MN) into the RV cavity, and the sheath is advanced slightly across the TV with some inferior deflection. Subsequently, the catheter is retroflexed using the D-curve creating a "reversed S-curve" on the whole system. The system is then gently pulled back, and the curve on the catheter is slowly opened to place the tip of the catheter just between the TV leaflet (anterior or septal) and the ventricular myocardium at the annulus. At this point, the Agilis curve is adjusted (closed/opened, moved clockwise/counterclockwise) to navigate between the leaflet and the ventricular wall.

INTRACAVITARY STRUCTURES

Intracavitary structures include the RV moderator band (MB) and the RV and LV papillary muscles.

ICE plays a particularly key role in mapping and ablation of these structures, as they cannot be visualized by fluoroscopy and are not easily represented on electroanatomic mapping.

The MB is a prominent muscular trabeculation that extends from the interventricular septum to the anterolateral wall of the RV and provides support to the anterior papillary muscle of the TV.[21] It can be visualized by advancing the ICE probe into the RV and then releasing flexion (**Fig. 11**A). Clockwise rotation allows visualization of the MB septal insertion, while counterclockwise rotation moves the imaging plane toward the free-wall insertion.

The 2 LV papillary muscles are termed ALPM and posteromedial (PMPM). They originate from the mid or apical third of the LV and give rise to multiple chordae tendinae, which attach to the MV leaflets.[22] The ALPM originates from the anterolateral LV wall and provides chordae to the

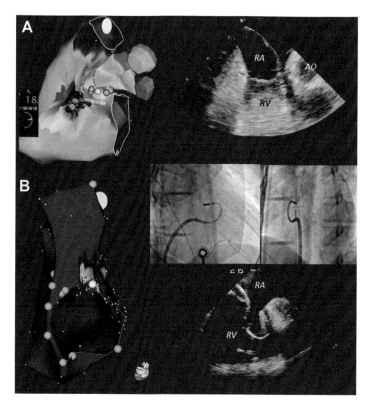

Fig. 9. Para-Hisian and TV VAs. (*A*) Ablation of para-Hisian PVC; the left panel shows a CARTOSOUND map demonstrating the relationship between the site of PVC elimination (*red dots*) and the sites with His electrograms (*yellow dots*); the right panel shows an ICE home view with the ablation catheter and the radiofrequency lesions (*red dots*). (*B*) Ablation of PVC from the superior tricuspid annulus using a "reversed S-curve" approach; electroanatomic map, right anterior oblique and left anterior oblique radiographic views, and ICE image are shown.

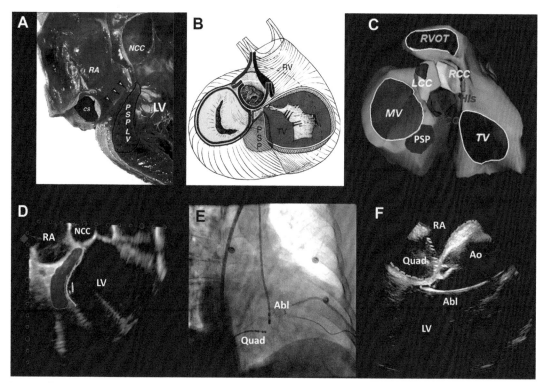

Fig. 10. The posterior superior process of the LV (PSPLV). (*A*) Anatomic preparation showing the relationship between the inferior RA, NCC, and the PSPLV. (*B, C*) Anatomic description and CARTOSOUND reconstruction showing the location of this region. (*D*) ICE view of the PSPLV obtained from the RA. (*E, F*) Case of idiopathic PVC ablated from the PSPLV via retrograde aortic approach; a quadripolar catheter is positioned at the His region. Abl, ablation catheter; Quad, quadripolar catheter. Image courtesy Dr. Luis Saenz.

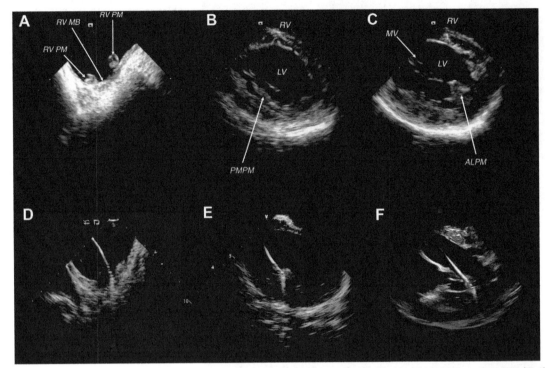

Fig. 11. Intracavitary structures. (*A–C*) ICE imaging of the MB and RV papillary muscles, PMPM, and ALPM. (*D–F*) Examples of PVC ablation showing the usefulness of ICE to assess catheter-tissue contact in each of these structures. PM, papillary muscle; PMPM, posteromedial papillary muscle.

anterolateral half of the anterior and posterior mitral leaflets. The PMPM originates from the inferoseptal LV wall and provides chordae to the posteromedial half of both leaflets. To visualize the LV papillary muscles, further clockwise rotation is applied from the RV view[23] (see **Fig. 11**B, C). This produces a long-axis view of the LV with the PMPM, which in most cases contains 2 or 3 heads or muscle groups. Additional clockwise torque brings into view the ALPM, which typically has a single head or muscle group.

ICE is useful to verify that the tip of the mapping/ablation catheter is in contact with the mapped structure instead of the ventricular free wall (see **Fig. 11**D–F). This is key to avoid "steam pops" in the free wall resulting in cardiac tamponade, especially if the ablation catheter is wedged between a papillary muscle and the ventricular wall.

SUMMARY

By allowing real-time definition of the cardiac anatomy and localization of catheters, ICE has become an invaluable tool for ablation of VAs. Its role is especially important in the anatomically complex outflow tract region, where many structures overlap in a relatively small area, and for ablation of intracavitary structures, which are not visualized by fluoroscopy.

REFERENCES

1. Cronin EM, Bogun FM, Maury P, et al. 2019 HRS/EHRA/APHRS/LAHRS expert consensus statement on catheter ablation of ventricular arrhythmias. Heart Rhythm 2020;17(1):e2–154.
2. Enriquez A, Saenz LC, Rosso R, et al. Use of intracardiac echocardiography in interventional cardiology: working with the anatomy rather than fighting it. Circulation 2018;137(21):2278–94.
3. Tanawuttiwat T, Nazarian S, Calkins H. The role of catheter ablation in the management of ventricular tachycardia. Eur Heart J 2016;37(7):594–609.
4. Liao Z, Zhan X, Wu S, et al. Idiopathic ventricular arrhythmias originating from the pulmonary sinus cusp: prevalence, electrocardiographic/electrophysiological characteristics, and catheter ablation. J Am Coll Cardiol 2015;66(23):2633–44.
5. Zhang J, Tang C, Zhang Y, et al. Pulmonary sinus cusp mapping and ablation: a new concept and approach for idiopathic right ventricular outflow tract arrhythmias. Heart Rhythm 2018;15(1):38–45.
6. Tabatabaei N, Asirvatham SJ. Supravalvular arrhythmia: identifying and ablating the substrate. Circ Arrhythm Electrophysiol 2009;2(3):316–26.

7. Sánchez-Quintana D, Doblado-Calatrava M, Cabrera JA, et al. Anatomical basis for the cardiac interventional electrophysiologist. Biomed Res Int 2015;2015:547364.

8. Futyma P, Moroka K, Derndorfer M, et al. Left pulmonary cusp ablation of refractory ventricular arrhythmia originating from the inaccessible summit. Europace 2019;21(8):1253.

9. Ehdaie A, Liu F, Cingolani E, et al. How to use intracardiac echocardiography to guide catheter ablation of outflow tract ventricular arrhythmias. Heart Rhythm 2020;17(8):1405–10.

10. Yang Y, Liu Q, Liu Z, et al. Treatment of pulmonary sinus cusp-derived ventricular arrhythmia with reversed U-curve catheter ablation. J Cardiovasc Electrophysiol 2017;28(7):768–75.

11. McAlpine WA. Heart and coronary arteries: an anatomical atlas for clinical diagnosis, radiological investigation, and surgical treatment. New York: Springer-Verlag; 1975.

12. Piazza N, de Jaegere P, Schultz C, et al. Anatomy of the aortic valvar complex and its implications for transcatheter implantation of the aortic valve. Circ Cardiovasc Interv 2008;1(1):74–81.

13. de Kerchove L, El Khoury G. Anatomy and pathophysiology of the ventriculo-aortic junction: implication in aortic valve repair surgery. Ann Cardiothorac Surg 2013;2(1):57–64.

14. Bala R, Garcia FC, Hutchinson MD, et al. Electrocardiographic and electrophysiologic features of ventricular arrhythmias originating from the right/left coronary cusp commissure. Heart Rhythm 2010; 7(3):312–22.

15. Roberts-Thomson KC, Steven D, Seiler J, et al. Coronary artery injury due to catheter ablation in adults:

presentations and outcomes. Circulation 2009; 120(15):1465–73.

16. Enriquez A, Tapias C, Rodriguez D, et al. How to map and ablate parahisian ventricular arrhythmias. Heart Rhythm 2018;15(8):1268–74.

17. Santangeli P, Hutchinson MD, Supple GE, et al. Right atrial approach for ablation of ventricular arrhythmias arising from the left posterior-superior process of the left ventricle. Circ Arrhythm Electrophysiol 2016;9(7):e004048.

18. Santangeli P, Hyman MC, Muser D, et al. Outcomes of percutaneous trans-right atrial access to the left ventricle for catheter ablation of ventricular tachycardia in patients with mechanical aortic and mitral valves. JAMA Cardiol 2020. https://doi.org/10. 1001/jamacardio.2020.4414.

19. Dahou A, Levin D, Reisman M, et al. Anatomy and physiology of the tricuspid valve. JACC Cardiovasc Imaging 2019;12(3):458–68.

20. Enriquez A, Tapias C, Rodriguez D, et al. Role of intracardiac echocardiography for guiding ablation of tricuspid valve arrhythmias. Heartrhythm Case Rep 2018;4(6):209–13.

21. Sadek MM, Benhayon D, Sureddi R, et al. Idiopathic ventricular arrhythmias originating from the moderator band: electrocardiographic characteristics and treatment by catheter ablation. Heart Rhythm 2015;12(1):67–75.

22. Roberts WC, Cohen LS. Left ventricular papillary muscles. Description of the normal and a survey of conditions causing them to be abnormal. Circulation 1972;46(1):138–54.

23. Enriquez A, Supple GE, Marchlinski FE, et al. How to map and ablate papillary muscle ventricular arrhythmias. Heart Rhythm 2017;14(11):1721–8.

Utility of Intracardiac Echocardiography for Guiding Ablation of Ventricular Tachycardia in Nonischemic Cardiomyopathy

Christopher Barrett, MD, Wendy S. Tzou, MD, FHRS*

KEYWORDS

- Intracardiac echocardiography • Ventricular tachycardia • Radiofrequency catheter • Ablation
- Nonischemic cardiomyopathy

KEY POINTS

- Intracardiac echocardiography (ICE) is a valuable tool for identifying structures that are difficult to access or adjacent to high-risk regions that are sensitive to damage from radiofrequency ablation.
- ICE can be used to ensure catheter position and stability during radiofrequency catheter ablation.
- ICE can be a useful adjunctive tool for targeting regions for ablation by identifying wall motion abnormalities, muscular hypertrophy, thrombus, and endocardial, midmyocardial, or epicardial scar.

 Video content accompanies this article at http://www.cardiacep.theclinics.com.

INTRODUCTION

Catheter ablation is an effective means for managing ventricular tachycardia (VT) in patients with structural heart disease, especially when medications have failed.[1] The primary mechanism for VT in such patients is reentry within regions of fibrosis or scar; such areas can be identified in the absence of ongoing VT, using intracardiac mapping or cardiac imaging.[1–3]

Uniformly acquiring preprocedural cardiac imaging in all patients is often not practically or clinically feasible, however, and additional challenges exist in ensuring adequate image acquisition and registration within the electroanatomic mapping (EAM) system for the purpose of guiding ablation. Understanding location of substrate is especially important when considering VT ablation in patients with nonischemic cardiomyopathy (NICM), as the

substrate is often epicardial or midmyocardial, both of which are often harder to identify with standard intracardiac mapping techniques and can add additional time and complexity to cases.[4,5] Intracardiac echocardiography (ICE) has emerged as an important adjunct, along with EAM, for real-time image and data acquisition in VT ablation procedures, particularly for NICM.[1,6,7]

The primary purpose of this article is to characterize findings on ICE, which can identify or confirm targets for ablation of ventricular arrhythmias. In addition, ways in which ICE can be used to improve procedural success in patients with NICM and ventricular arrhythmias, including premature ventricular contractions (PVCs), and review of current consensus guidelines regarding the use of ICE for guidance of VT ablation are discussed.

Division of Cardiology, Section of Cardiac Electrophysiology, University of Colorado School of Medicine Anschutz Medical Campus, Aurora, CO, USA
* Corresponding author. 12401 East 17th Avenue, MS B-136, Aurora, CO 80045.
E-mail address: Wendy.tzou@cuanschutz.edu

Card Electrophysiol Clin 13 (2021) 337–343
https://doi.org/10.1016/j.ccep.2021.03.008
1877-9182/21/© 2021 Elsevier Inc. All rights reserved.

IMAGE ACQUISITION

Phased-array catheters, as opposed to rotational or radial ICE catheters, are preferred for use in ablation procedures, given better image resolution at greater depths, as well as relative maneuverability and versatility.[7] The additional ability to incorporate multiple 2-dimensional slices into a 3-dimensional (3D) reconstruction within the EAM system, which is currently only possible with the CARTO EAM system (Biosense Webster, Diamond Bar, CA, USA), makes it particularly attractive for use in defining anatomy and identifying substrate in complex ablations.

In addition to characterizing baseline anatomy, ICE is an invaluable tool for verifying appropriate catheter position, and especially when navigating or attempting to stabilize the catheter on intracavitary structures, such as the papillary muscles or right ventricle (RV) moderator band, or structures that are otherwise difficult to visualize fluoroscopically, including the pulmonary valve, aortic root, coronary cusps, and even the ostia of the coronary arteries.[7,8]

Descriptions about how to acquire images of the ventricles from either the right atrium (RA) or the RV have been detailed in previous articles and will not be discussed specifically here except to emphasize that images of the main body of the left ventricle (LV) or left ventricular outflow tract (LVOT) and aortic root are typically obtained most clearly with the transducer positioned within the RV. Depending on anatomy, however, alternative views of the LV and LVOT may also be acquired from the RA.

UTILITY OF INTRACARDIAC ECHOCARDIOGRAPHY IN IDENTIFYING REENTRANT VENTRICULAR TACHYCARDIA SUBSTRATE IN NONISCHEMIC CARDIOMYOPATHY

Arrhythmogenic substrate in NICM generally localizes to perivalvular regions.[9,10] In the case of VT involving the LV free wall or septum, ICE signs indicating the likely presence of midmyocardial or epicardial tissue include localized hyperechogenicity, with or without associated wall motion abnormality, which persists after decreasing the gain on the ultrasound system in order to exclude noise[11] (Fig. 1A, B). In the seminal study demonstrating the utility of ICE in identifying epicardial substrate in NICM VT patients, Bala and colleagues[11] demonstrated this signature finding in the annular, lateral LV in 18 patients, all of whom had abnormal epicardial substrate confirmed with subsequent EAM; none of the 30 control

patients with structurally normal hearts demonstrated this ICE finding. Such increased echogenicity has subsequently been correlated with endocardial unipolar voltage abnormalities as well as with regions of late gadolinium enhancement on cardiac MRI, thus verifying its significance when identified[7,11,12] (Fig. 1).

ICE can also be helpful in quickly identifying nonischemic substrate (and therefore alter the mapping and ablation strategy) in an increasingly observed population of patients with a history of ischemic heart disease and who are thought to have ischemic VT.[13] The scar distribution owing to prior myocardial infarction typically extends from the endocardium to midmyocardium to epicardium, and not vice versa. Observing an inverse pattern of scar distribution, specifically one that involves only the epicardium or midmyocardium and not the endocardium, is inconsistent with postinfarction substrate and suggests the presence of at least a mixed cardiomyopathy, even if the patient has a history of prior myocardial infarction[12] (Fig. 2).

Importantly, this substrate information can be quickly acquired at the outset of the case and can instruct whether (1) epicardial access for mapping and ablation should ensue, or (2) use of alternative radiofrequency (RF) ablation techniques, including hypotonic irrigant or bipolar ablation, which can produce deeper or more transmural RF lesions,[12] should be considered.[14]

UTILITY OF INTRACARDIAC ECHOCARDIOGRAPHY IN MAPPING AND ABLATION OF VENTRICULAR ARRHYTHMIAS IN NONISCHEMIC CARDIOMYOPATHY

Once baseline images are acquired, ICE can help to guide mode, as well as safety of access, and especially when transseptal access to the LV is planned.[3] After access is obtained, the positions of catheter or catheters and long sheaths can be directly visualized throughout the duration of the case, and vigilance to monitoring for complications, including thrombus formation, cardiac perforation, and pericardial effusion, is enhanced.[14,15]

When CARTOSOUND ICE (Biosense Webster, Diamond Bar, CA, USA) is used with the CARTO mapping system, not only can ICE-acquired images of basic anatomic structures be reconstructed 3-dimensionally[7,8] but ICE images of substrate or scar (hyperechogenic regions) can also be incorporated into the 3D map (see Fig. 1). Obvious advantages of such real-time image acquisition and integration include the ability to target substrate with reduced need for fluoroscopy and without need for alternative, resource-

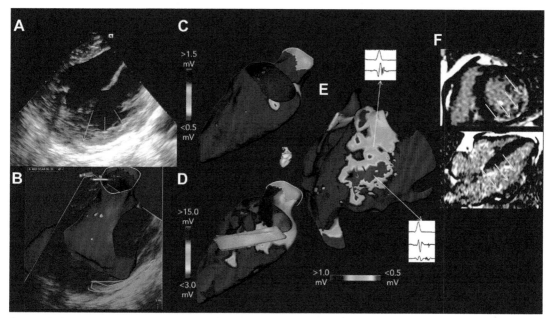

Fig. 1. ICE images with example of integration of ICE images within the EAM system (*A, B*), electroanatomic voltage maps (*C–E*), and cardiac MRI (*F*) from a patient with NICM and VT. The posterolateral projection of. the endocardial LV bipolar voltage map (*C*) demonstrates no significant LV endocardial abnormality. However, real-time ICE images (*A*) demonstrate a hyperechoic region (*orange arrows*) in the inferolateral midmyocardium to epicardium consistent with fibrotic substrate; in the CARTO system, 2-dimensional contours of the region of interest (*B*) are collected and integrated into the 3D EAM (*D*, reconstructed 3D scar location using ICE contours collected at different LV angles). Note that the scar location as seen on ICE correlates with the region of unipolar voltage abnormality in the inferolateral, perimitral annular midmyocardium to epicardium (*D*). In this case, the threshold for abnormal unipolar voltage was increased, which uncovered the deeper substrate. The presence of true epicardial substrate in the same regions identified on ICE and unipolar voltage mapping was then confirmed with epicardial access and bipolar voltage mapping, revealing low-voltage regions with late potentials and abnormal local conduction (*E*). Cardiac MRI demonstrates late gadolinium enhancement (*yellow arrows*) in the same regions as those observed on intraprocedural mapping and ICE.

intensive, preprocedural imaging and associated errors introduced with merging of images with the EAM.[1] If epicardial mapping and ablation are indicated, ICE can then be used to guide safe percutaneous epicardial access, as the guidewire passed through can be easily visualized to confirm proper location within the pericardial space, as opposed to within the RV.

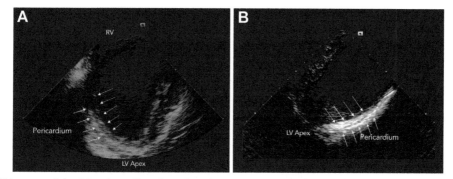

Fig. 2. ICE images of the LV endocardium from 2 patients presenting with VT: (*A*) patient A had a history of prior anterior myocardial infarction, and (*B*) patient B had a history of inferior myocardial infarction but mixed cardiomyopathy as substrate for VT. Note the difference in scar distribution, as identified by hyperechogenicity on ICE (*white arrows*) between patients. Patient A has findings consistent with postinfarction VT, with scar extending from endocardium to midmyocardium, with associated wall thinning and dyskinesis. Patient B's substrate distribution is predominantly midmyocardial and epicardial.

Among patients undergoing repeated ablation attempt, ICE is of particular value. In a cohort of 88 patients with NICM and ventricular arrhythmias undergoing repeat ablation at the University of Colorado, ICE was essential in identifying midmyocardial or epicardial substrate in 20%; those patients with midmyocardial substrate often required multiple repeated ablation attempts targeting identified substrate, and approximately one-third required use of adjunctive techniques to enhance depth of RF ablation lesions to subsequently lead to durable arrhythmia control.[12]

The utility of ICE, especially with ICE-image integration, in refining ablation of ventricular arrhythmias arising from papillary muscles was nicely described by Proietti and colleagues,[8] among a series of 16 patients with frequent PVCs or VT with cardiomyopathy. In their series, detailed geometries of the LV and papillary muscles at the outset of the cases permitted mapping information to be localized more accurately to the papillary muscles themselves (rather than being interpolated imprecisely within the LV endocardium) as well as helped to confirm catheter stability on the body of the papillary muscles during ablation. This ICE-facilitated 3D EAM approach resulted in intermediate-term lack of ventricular arrhythmia recurrence in 87.5%, which compares favorably to success rates of 60% reported in longer-term follow-up of patients undergoing papillary muscle PVC ablations.[16] Similar approaches have been used with success in ablation of PVCs or VT arising from the LVOT and periaortic region[7,17,18]

ADDITIONAL INTRACARDIAC ECHOCARDIOGRAPHY UTILITIES

Wall motion abnormalities, such as regions of ventricular akinesia or dyskinesia, in patients with VT are classically associated with ischemic cardiomyopathy. However, focal ventricular abnormalities may be identifiable in select patients with nonischemic causes of VT, which can be useful for initial mapping of fragmented and middiastolic potentials during ablation procedures. In 2004, Jongbloed and colleagues[19] incorporated ICE imaging to identify focal ventricular aneurysms to help target sites for ablation in patients with arrhythmogenic right ventricular cardiomyopathy. Similarly, ICE was able to identify areas of marked septal hypertrophy corresponding with early fragmented signals during VT in patients with hypertrophic obstructive cardiomyopathy (HOCM).

In addition to detecting normal and abnormal myocardium, ICE can also be a useful tool for real-time detection of intracardiac thrombus. Although the transesophageal echocardiogram is principally used to detect atrial thrombi for procedures such as direct current cardioversion and left atrial appendage occlusion device placement, ICE has been described as a tool with increased sensitivity for identification of ventricular thrombus before proceeding with endocardial ablation.[20] In 2016, Peichl and colleagues[20] published a case series of 8 patients with drug-refractory VT in whom mural, chronic LV thrombus was detected by transthoracic or ICE. VT ablations were then performed with ICE, which allowed delineation of thrombus borders and guided endocardial catheter manipulations and ablation, and no clinically apparent embolic events were subsequently observed.[20] Conversely, presence of nonlaminated, nonmural, or mobile thrombus can also be observed on ICE before access to the left cardiac chambers, especially when transthoracic images are limited (**Fig. 3**, Video 1); in that instance, and in the absence of an urgent or emergent need, catheter ablation should be avoided until a sufficient period of anticoagulation and reassessment for interval resolution has been allowed.[1]

Finally, ICE enables the ability to confirm catheter contact and to observe real-time ablation lesion formation as well as for excessive heating and potential for steam pop, especially when using adjunctive techniques to enhance RF lesion size (**Fig. 4**, Video 2).[21]

CONSIDERATIONS

Although ICE is an important tool for real-time assessment of intracardiac structures and anatomic relationships, there are some limitations to consider with regards to its use in VT ablation procedures. Image quality may vary depending on patient anatomy and tissue-specific characteristics, the resolution of which may be further degraded in the presence of multiple other sheaths, catheters, or intracardiac devices, which can produce shadowing artifact, or simply be in the field of view of the transducer, thus obscuring and distorting image quality. Some of these factors can be potentially mitigated by imaging from the vantage point of the pericardial sinuses, using the transcutaneous access obtained for epicardial mapping and ablation of NICM VT; however, the need for intrapericardial access and manipulation, and potentially increased risk associated, limits its use to specific circumstances and more experienced operators.[22] Outside of intrapericardial imaging, additional venous access is typically required when ICE is used, which can incrementally increase the risk of vascular-related complications. Cost is also an important potential limitation, which is a significant reason accounting

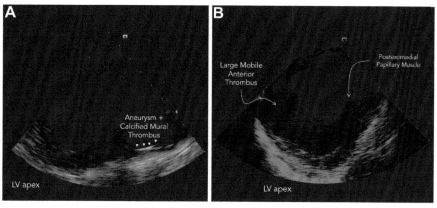

Fig. 3. Thrombus evaluation with ICE. (*A*) A calcified, chronic thrombus (*arrowheads*) within an LV posterobasal aneurysm. (*B*) A large anterior LV thrombus is demonstrated, distinct from the posteromedial as well as anterolateral (not shown) papillary muscles.

for less frequent adoption at centers outside of the United States.[23]

EXPERT CONSENSUS RECOMMENDATIONS

Despite the widespread use of ICE for ablation of VT in patients with NICM, there is a paucity of consensus guidelines regarding its standard use for these procedures. In 2009, the American Society of Echocardiography released guidelines regarding echocardiography-guided interventions; the usefulness of ICE for locating anatomic structures, guiding transseptal puncture, monitoring lesion formation, and monitoring for complications during ablation procedures was recognized, although the concrete recommendations provided were limited to its use in guiding transseptal puncture and monitoring aspects of pulmonary vein isolation for atrial fibrillation.[24]

The 2019, HRS/EHRA/APHRS/LAHRS Expert Consensus Statement on VT ablation formally recognized the importance of ICE in multiple facets of ventricular arrhythmia ablation, including as a means to better define intracavitary structures and papillary muscles, as a tool for early recognition of procedural complications, including pericardial effusion, and for identification of segments of myocardium with wall thinning, wall motion abnormalities, increased echogenicity, and mural thrombus.[1]

SUMMARY AND RECOMMENDED APPROACH

Phased-array ICE is a valuable imaging adjunct for guiding VT ablation in patients with NICM. For patients with VT originating in the LV, the ICE catheter is most frequently positioned in the RV for optimal visualization of structures on the left. During ablation procedures for NICM, ICE can be

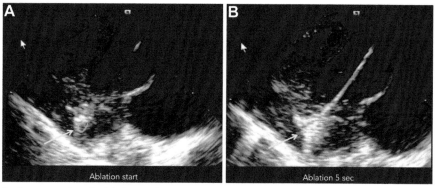

Fig. 4. ICE findings associated with impending steam pop during RF ablation. Note the rapid rate of increased echogenicity of the LV at the ablation catheter tip–tissue interface as well as increased formation of bubbles within the blood pool on ICE (*A*) from the initiation of open-irrigated RF ablation to (*B*) 5 seconds after application using 50 W. (Figure reproduced with permission from Catheter Ablation of Catheter Arrhythmias, 4th ed. Eds. Huang and Miller, Elsevier: Philadelphia, 2020.)

routinely used for obtaining transseptal access, guiding catheter position, and ensuring catheter stability around structures, such as papillary muscles, valves, and coronary arteries. ICE is an invaluable tool for rapidly identifying epicardial or midmyocardial scar that can be substrate for VT, which can be more difficult to identify using endocardial EAM techniques. Rapid identification of nonischemic substrate using ICE can save time at the initiation of ablation procedures and guide upfront, targeted VT ablation strategy. Furthermore, ICE can improve the safety of VT ablation by clearly identifying intracardiac thrombus and monitoring for real-time complications, such as steam pop, catheter thrombus, or cardiac perforation.

CLINICS CARE POINTS

- Intracardiac echocardiography is routinely used during ventricular tachycardia ablation procedures for obtaining transseptal access and ensuring catheter position around structures of interest.

- Intracardiac echocardiography can be used to quickly identify substrate for nonischemic ventricular tachycardia, such as epicardial or midmyocardial scar, ventricular aneurysm, or muscular hypertrophy

- Intracardiac echocardiography can be used to confirm catheter location and stability during mapping and ablation as well as to monitor acute ablation effect.

- Intracardiac echocardiography can be used to monitor in real-time for procedural complications of ventricular tachycardia ablation, including catheter thrombus formation, steam pop, and cardiac perforation.

RELEVANT DISCLOSURES

Dr W.S. Tzou has received speaker honoraria or is a consultant for Abbott, Biosense Webster, Boston Scientific, Biotronik, BioSig, and Medtronic and research funding from Abbott, Biosense Webster, and Boston Scientific. Dr C. Barrett has no relevant disclosures.

SUPPLEMENTARY DATA

Supplementary data related to this article can be found online at https://doi.org/10.1016/j.ccep.2021.03.008.

REFERENCES

1. Cronin EM, Bogun FM, Maury P, et al. 2019 HRS/EHRA/APHRS/LAHRS expert consensus statement on catheter ablation of ventricular arrhythmias: executive summary. Heart Rhythm 2019;17(1):e155–205.
2. Soto-Iglesias D, Penela D, Jauregui B, et al. Cardiac magnetic resonance-guided ventricular tachycardia substrate ablation. JACC Clin Electrophysiol 2020;6: 436–47.
3. Takigawa M, Duchateau J, Sacher F, et al. Are wall thickness channels defined by computed tomography predictive of isthmuses of postinfarction ventricular tachycardia? Heart Rhythm 2019;16:1661–8.
4. Muser D, Liang JJ, Pathak RK, et al. Long-term outcomes of catheter ablation of electrical storm in nonischemic dilated cardiomyopathy compared with ischemic cardiomyopathy. JACC Clin Electrophysiol 2017;3:767–78.
5. Nakahara S, Tung R, Ramirez RJ, et al. Characterization of the arrhythmogenic substrate in ischemic and nonischemic cardiomyopathy: implications for catheter ablation of hemodynamically unstable ventricular tachycardia. J Am Coll Cardiol 2010;55: 2355–65.
6. Ren JF, Marchlinski FE. Intracardiac echocardiography imaging in radiofrequency catheter ablation for ventricular tachycardia. In: Ren JF, Marchlinski FE, Callans DJ, et al, editors. Practical intracardiac echocardiography in electrophysiology. Malden (MA): Blackwell Publishing; 2006. p. 150–67.
7. Enriquez A, Saenz LC, Rosso R, et al. Use of intracardiac echocardiography in interventional cardiology: working with the anatomy rather than fighting it. Circulation 2018;137:2278–94.
8. Proietti R, Rivera S, Dussault C, et al. Intracardiac echo-facilitated 3D electroanatomical mapping of ventricular arrhythmias from the papillary muscles: assessing the 'fourth dimension' during ablation. Europace 2017;19:21–8.
9. Cano O, Hutchinson M, Lin D, et al. Electroanatomic substrate and ablation outcome for suspected epicardial ventricular tachycardia in left ventricular nonischemic cardiomyopathy. J Am Coll Cardiol 2009;54:799–808.
10. Nakajima I, Narui R, Aboud AA, et al. Periaortic ventricular tachycardias in nonischemic cardiomyopathy: substrate and electrocardiographic correlations. Circ Arrhythm Electrophysiol 2021; 14(2):e008887.
11. Bala R, Ren JF, Hutchinson MD, et al. Assessing epicardial substrate using intracardiac echocardiography during VT ablation. Circ Arrhythm Electrophysiol 2011;4:667–73.
12. Tzou WS, Rothstein PA, Cowherd M, et al. Repeat ablation of refractory ventricular arrhythmias in patients with nonischemic cardiomyopathy: impact of

midmyocardial substrate and role of adjunctive ablation techniques. J Cardiovasc Electrophysiol 2018;29:1403–12.

13. Aldhoon B, Tzou WS, Riley MP, et al. Nonischemic cardiomyopathy substrate and ventricular tachycardia in the setting of coronary artery disease. Heart Rhythm 2013;10:1622–7.

14. Ren JF, Marchlinski FE. Utility of intracardiac echocardiography in left heart ablation for tachyarrhythmias. Echocardiography 2007;24:533–40.

15. Filgueiras-Rama D, de Torres-Alba F, Castrejon-Castrejon S, et al. Utility of intracardiac echocardiography for catheter ablation of complex cardiac arrhythmias in a medium-volume training center. Echocardiography 2015;32:660–70.

16. Latchamsetty R, Yokokawa M, Morady F, et al. Multicenter outcomes for catheter ablation of idiopathic premature ventricular complexes. J Am Coll Cardiol 2015;1:116–23.

17. Hutchinson MD, Garcia FC. An organized approach to the localization, mapping, and ablation of outflow tract ventricular arrhythmias. J Cardiovasc Electrophysiol 2013;24:1189–97.

18. Lamberti F, Calo L, Pandozi C, et al. Radiofrequency catheter ablation of idiopathic left ventricular outflow tract tachycardia: utility of intracardiac echocardiography. J Cardiovasc Electrophysiol 2001;12:529–35.

19. Jongbloed MR, Bax JJ, van der Burg AE, et al. Radiofrequency catheter ablation of ventricular tachycardia guided by intracardiac echocardiography. Eur J Echocardiogr 2004;5:34–40.

20. Peichl P, Wichterle D, Cihak R, et al. Catheter ablation of ventricular tachycardia in the presence of an old endocavitary thrombus guided by intracardiac echocardiography. Pacing Clin Electrophysiol 2016;39:581–7.

21. Nguyen DT, Zipse M, Borne RT, et al. Use of tissue electric and ultrasound characteristics to predict and prevent steam-generated cavitation during high-power radiofrequency ablation. JACC Clin Electrophysiol 2018;4:491–500.

22. Horowitz BN, Vaseghi M, Mahajan A, et al. Percutaneous intrapericardial echocardiography during catheter ablation: a feasibility study. Heart Rhythm 2006;3:1275–82.

23. Basman C, Parmar YJ, Kronzon I. Intracardiac echocardiography for structural heart and electrophysiological interventions. Curr Cardiol Rep 2017;19:102.

24. Silvestry FE, Kerber RE, Brook MM, et al. Echocardiography-guided interventions. J Am Soc Echocardiography 2009;22:213–31 [quiz: 316–7].

Intracardiac Echocardiography to Guide Mapping and Ablation of Arrhythmias in Patients with Congenital Heart Disease

Timothy Campbell, BSc[a,b], Haris Haqqani, MD, PhD[c],
Saurabh Kumar, BSc(Med), MBBS, PhD[a,b],*

KEYWORDS

- Congenital heart disease • Cardiac abnormality • Arrhythmia • Intracardiac echocardiography

KEY POINTS

- ICE is complimentary to fluoroscopy during ablation for real-time assessment of ablation catheter position and to potentially minimize prolonged ionizing radiation exposure in younger patients.
- Complex anatomic reconstructions associated with repaired CHD, areas of wall thickening, inaccessible regions caused by suture lines, baffles, and conduits can all be visualized in real time with ICE.
- ICE imaging positions in patients with CHD are consistent with standard imaging approaches from the RA, RV, or CS, except when atrial or ventricular reconstructed anatomy is present.
- ICE guidance is safe and effective when per- forming a transbaffle/transconduit puncture.

INTRODUCTION

Congenital heart disease (CHD) encompasses a range of structural cardiac abnormalities present before birth that are attributable to abnormal fetal cardiac development.[1] The global prevalence of CHD has been estimated to be nearly 1.8% of births.[2] Surgical advancements in CHD have improved survival from the first year of life to greater than 90% into adulthood.[3] Although surgical intervention has improved survival, almost all patients with adult CHD have sequelae related to their underlying CHD or its repair or palliation.[1] Complex arrhythmias are a common cause of morbidity in the adult CHD population, with estimates of approximately 50% of 20-year-olds with CHD developing an atrial tachyarrhythmia during their lifetimes.[4] Sinoatrial dysfunction, atrioventricular block, and ventricular and supraventricular tachyarrhythmias are common.[4] Congenital abnormalities prone to arrhythmias include Ebstein anomaly, transposition of the great arteries, tricuspid atresia, pulmonary atresia, hypoplastic left heart syndrome, septal defects, heterotaxy, and tetralogy of Fallot.[5] The complete range of tachyarrhythmias have all been reported, including atrial fibrillation, atrioventricular reentrant tachycardia (AVRT), atrioventricular nodal reentrant tachycardia (AVNRT), focal atrial tachycardia, intra-atrial reentry (IART), and ventricular tachycardia (VT).[5,6]

Improved survival among patients with CHD is leading to a growing population of adults with

[a] Department of Cardiology, Westmead Hospital, Sydney, Australia; [b] Westmead Applied Research Centre, University of Sydney, New South Wales, Australia; [c] Prince Charles Hospital, University of Queensland, Brisbane, Qld, Australia
* Corresponding author. Department of Cardiology, Westmead Hospital, Westmead Applied Research Centre, University of Sydney, Darcy Road, Westmead, New South Wales 2145, Australia.
E-mail address: saurabh.kumar@sydney.edu.au

Card Electrophysiol Clin 13 (2021) 345–356
https://doi.org/10.1016/j.ccep.2021.03.001

highly complex postrepair anatomy that can be prone to arrhythmias. Because of their young age, antiarrhythmic drug therapy is challenging, requiring extended periods of drug therapy with the potential risk of proarrhythmia and side effects.[4] Catheter ablation therefore is an increasingly viable option for these patients but requires a comprehensive understanding of the surgical intervention for appropriate procedural planning. Preprocedural imaging via computed tomography (CT) or MRI can be used for planning and integration to guide ablation. In addition, procedures can be enhanced by the use of intracardiac echocardiography (ICE), which provides unrivalled real-time visualization of anatomic structures critical in these procedures. In addition, ICE is able to visualize repaired cardiac suture lines, baffles, and conduits.[4,7] It also allows assessment of catheter contact, monitoring lesion formation, and rapid diagnosis of complications. This article describes the role of ICE in catheter ablation procedures for arrhythmias in CHD.

INTRACARDIAC ECHOCARDIOGRAPHIC IMAGING

Initial experience with ICE in CHD was used to guide percutaneous device closure of atrial septal defects and patent foramen ovale.[8] As experience has grown with ICE, use for identification of complex anatomic features critical to arrhythmias has improved. ICE offers several benefits for ablation procedures in general but also for patients with CHD (**Box 1**). In general, ICE provides real-time visualization of catheter tip to tissue contact; monitoring for acute complications during atrial

---

Box 1
Benefits of intracardiac echocardiography in congenital heart disease

- Continuous live imaging
- Identification of complex anatomic features; for example, suture lines, baffles and conduits, wall thicknesses
- Catheter tip to tissue contact
- Lesion formation
- Monitoring for acute complications
- Use of Doppler to differentiate anatomic structures
- Enables shorter imaging distances[a]
- Provides higher resolution[a]

[a] Compared with transesophageal or transthoracic echocardiography.

---

and ventricular procedures; imaging of lesion morphologic changes that include swelling, dimpling, crater formation, accelerated bubbles formation, as a harbinger to a steam pop; and increased echogenicity during/immediately after lesion deployment.[9,10] Use of Doppler with the ICE probe also enables accurate identification of relevant anatomic structures, including baffles, conduits, vascular structures, and main cardiac chambers.[4] A broad appreciation of real-time cardiac structures in CHD is invaluable when navigating the complex anatomy.[11]

Compared with transthoracic and transesophageal echocardiography (TEE), ICE imaging enables shorter imaging distances and higher resolution.[12] ICE provides complimentary real-time functional imaging of complex anatomy related to repaired CHD when integration of three-dimensional models reconstructed from CT or MRI are used in electroanatomic mapping (EAM) systems.

Septal Defects

The prevalence of septal defects ranges between 3% and 32% in the CHD population.[3] Arrhythmias related to septal defects are commonly related to surgical repair access sites via an atriotomy or ventriculotomy incision, or the septal patch.[13–15] However, the commonest reentrant tachycardia in this group overall remains cavotricuspid isthmus–dependent atrial flutter. ICE is helpful to identify, either by two-dimensional imaging or with color flow Doppler, the presence of a persistent foramen ovale, atrial septal defect (ASD), or ventricular septal defect (VSD). Surgically closed ASDs have an atriotomy performed in the lateral wall of the right atrium (RA), whereas repaired VSDs may have a ventriculotomy through the right ventricular outflow tract (RVOT). Imaging with ICE may be able to identify regions with increased echogenicity from the atriotomy by starting in the mid-RA and rotating counterclockwise to the free wall of the RA. Imaging of a VSD and/or ventriculotomy can be achieved from the RVOT. Counterclockwise rotation can view the free wall where the incision was created, and clockwise rotation interrogates the septum and the VSD region. Depending on the VSD location, positioning the ICE catheter near the septum may provide suboptimal views. Imaging away from the septum, from the low lateral RA or coronary sinus (CS), improves visualization of the interventricular septum (IVS; **Fig. 1**). Percutaneously closed ASDs may also have atrial arrhythmias and require access to the left atrium (LA). ICE can be used to guide transseptal puncture either away from the device or through the device.[16,17]

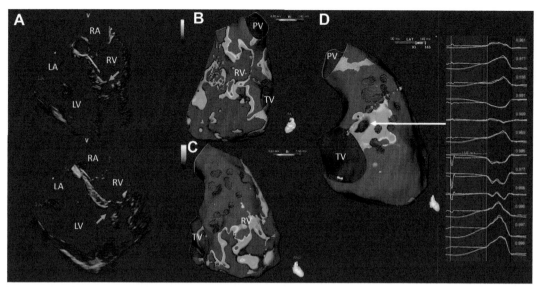

Fig. 1. VSD and VT. VSD on ICE, but unrelated to VT critical site. (*A*) VSD on ICE in mid to apical third of IVS. ICE catheter positioned in low lateral RA. (*B*) EAM reconstructions of bipolar voltage in posterior-anterior (PA) and (*C*) right anterior oblique (RAO) views. (*D*) EAM of late potentials and site of longest stimulus to QRS pace map with 97% correlation. LA, left atrium; LV, left ventricle; RV, right ventricle; TV, tricuspid valve.

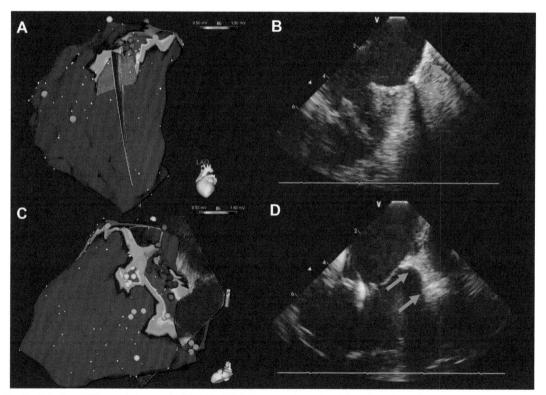

Fig. 2. RV after TOF repair imaged with ICE. (*A*) EAM reconstruction of RV bipolar voltage map in left anterior oblique (LAO) view. ICE catheter in the RVOT imaged through the anterior wall. Green reconstruction is of scar observed via ICE. (*B*) Corresponding ICE of RV anterior wall. Scar on ICE (*green arrows*). (*C*) EAM reconstruction of RV bipolar voltage map in posterior view shows low voltage from the pulmonary valve (PV) to the superior and septal TV. ICE catheter in the mid-RA imaged through the TV to the RV. (*D*) Corresponding ICE of RV. Scar on ICE (*green arrows*) at the superior TV. (Images courtesy of Dr Usha Tedrow, Brigham and Women's Hospital, MA, USA.)

Tetralogy of Fallot

Tetralogy of Fallot (TOF) is the commonest form of conotruncal CHD, with 4 morphologic features: pulmonary valve stenosis, VSD, an overriding aorta, and right ventricular hypertrophy. It occurs in 0.023% to 0.063% of live births and accounts for 8% to 10% of the CHD population.[3,18] Surgical correction repairs the pulmonary stenosis and VSD and may require an incision through the free wall of the right ventricle (RV) outflow tract in addition to transatrial and transpulmonary artery approaches. The prevalence of atrial and ventricular arrhythmias after repair is estimated to be 20% and 15% respectively, with rapid increases after 45 years of age.[1] Reentrant tachyarrhythmias in TOF may have critical circuit components in the isthmuses between anatomic boundaries of the pulmonary and tricuspid valves, VSD repair and ventriculotomy of the free wall of the RV,[14] or atriotomy in the RA. The substrate for ventricular arrhythmias may be visible with ICE at site of ventriculotomy and has increased echogenicity (**Fig. 2**). Imaging from the RA can delineate the superior tricuspid valve region isthmus. As discussed earlier, imaging from the RVOT can view the free wall of the RVOT where the incision was created, and clockwise rotation interrogates the septum and the VSD region, but imaging may be suboptimal depending on site of repair. Therefore, alternative imaging from the low lateral RA or CS can assist in visualization of the septum.

After Atrial Surgical Reconstruction

Fontan procedure as a result of tricuspid or pulmonary atresia

The Fontan procedure was first reported in 1971, enabling the direct drainage of the systemic venous circulation to the pulmonary circuit in patients with tricuspid or pulmonary atresia or functionally univentricular hearts. Varying approaches have been described depending on the anatomic reconstruction required, with the main types being (1) a direct connection of the atriopulmonary connection; (2) a lateral tunnel conduit of inferior vena caval drainage to the pulmonary artery; and (3) an extracardiac total cavopulmonary connection (TCPC).[19–22] Postrepair sinus node dysfunction and atrial arrhythmia risk is high, with up to 60% developing an atrial tachyarrhythmia.[3] Depending on the type of Fontan anatomy, an approach via a transbaffle or conduit puncture may be required if catheter ablation is undertaken[7,23] (**Fig. 3**). In the presence of a lateral tunnel or TCPC, careful and precise delineation of the conduit is required to access the arrhythmia substrate. ICE imaging may be difficult if peripheral vasculature is tortuous, if the patient has small vessels, or if a complete inferior vena cava

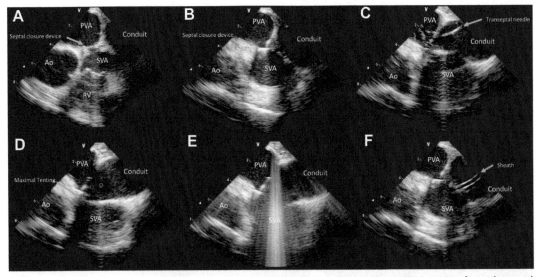

Fig. 3. Transconduit puncture in a Fontan circulation to the right Pulmonary Artery. ICE imaging from the esophagus. (*A*) Imaging from the esophagus visualizing through the conduit to the remnant systemic venous atrium (SVA), TV, and remnant RV. Septal closure device for an ASD between the remnant SVA and pulmonary venous atrium (PVA). (*B*) Clockwise rotation of ICE catheter shows more rightward extent of the closure device. (*C*) Puncture from conduit to PVA with contrast injection in PVA. (*D*) Tenting of the conduit to the remnant SVA. (*E*) Radiofrequency needle delivery for puncture from conduit to PVA at site of maximal tenting. (*F*) Postconduit puncture to SVA with sheath position. AO, aorta; PVA, pulmonary venous atrium. (Images courtesy of Drs John Triedman and Dominic Abrams, Boston Children's Hospital, MA, USA.)

(IVC) interruption or occlusion is present.[23] In this instance, use of the internal jugular vein or esophagus with the ICE catheter has been reported.[23,24] From the esophagus, ICE imaging can be performed with clockwise rotation to visualize more rightward anatomy and counterclockwise more leftward anatomy. Advancement of the probe shows more inferior structures, such as the cavotricuspid isthmus (**Fig. 4**). When imaging from the lateral tunnel or extracardiac conduit, ICE probe maneuverability may be reduced depending on the size of the chamber. If access to the systemic venous atrium (SVA) is routine, then imaging can be performed as in a structurally normal heart. Imaging an atriopulmonary connection requires either advancement to the approximate level of the anastomosis or a more inferior position with posterior deflection angling the beam through the superior SVA. Color Doppler

may also be helpful if identification of a remnant RV is required.

Atrial switch procedure to manage transposition of the great arteries

Transposition of the great arteries occurs in 0.02% to 0.03% of live births and in 1% to 7% of the CHD population.[3,25] The atrial switch procedure was developed in the mid–twentieth century and is an atrial reconstruction for establishment of durable communication of systemic and venous circulations in transposition of the great arteries.[26] An atrial switch uses either a synthetic material (Mustard) or the patient's own tissue (Senning) to redirect venous flow via an intra-atrial baffle to the appropriate ventricle. Sinus node dysfunction is the most common arrhythmia postprocedure, affecting approximately 48%, whereas atrial tachyarrhythmias occur in 13% to 30% of patients.[7] Intra-atrial

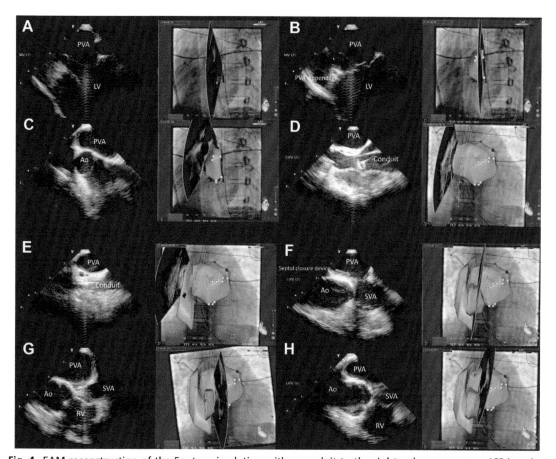

Fig. 4. EAM reconstruction of the Fontan circulation with a conduit to the right pulmonary artery. ICE imaging from the esophagus. (*A–E*) Clockwise rotation from mitral valve (MV) to the rightward extent of the conduit. (*Left*) ICE image and (*right*) corresponding catheter position in LAO and anterior-Posterior views. EAM reconstruction of PVA. White tags delineating MV. Light blue tags delineating edges of closure device between SVA and PVA. (*F and G*) Counterclockwise rotation through the conduit, SVA, and remnant RV. (Images courtesy of Drs John Triedman and Dominic Abrams, Boston Children's Hospital, MA, USA.)

reentry after surgical intervention can occur in a myriad of circuits but the most common is cavotricuspid isthmus (CTI)–dependent flutter. This condition is usually complicated by a component of the CTI being separated by the baffle, effectively creating 2 isthmuses, 1 between the tricuspid annulus and the baffle and a second from the baffle to the IVC.[7] Successful ablation requires therapy from both sides of the baffle for bidirectional conduction block. Access to the pulmonary venous atrium (PVA) can be achieved via a retrograde approach through the aorta and systemic RV but catheter stability can be difficult on the isthmus.[23] Depending on the anatomic reconstruction, a transbaffle puncture may be required.[7] Alternatively, there is a high incidence of baffle leaks in adults (up to 65% has been reported[27]) following atrial switch procedures, which may facilitate access for mapping and ablation catheter or as a site for arrhythmia (**Fig. 5**).

Imaging for intra-atrial reentrant tachycardia requires definition of both the SVA and PVA. Advancement into the SVA positions the catheter more leftward than in a structurally normal atrium because it follows the course of the SVA around the PVA. Counterclockwise rotation from the mitral valve visualizes the PVA and tricuspid valve. Slight withdrawal visualizes the SVA end of the CTI (**Fig. 6**).

Arterial Switch Procedure as Result of Transposition of the Great Arteries

The arterial switch procedure was first successfully performed by Jatene and coworkers in 1982.[26] As a result, the atrial tachyarrhythmias that occurred in older patients following atrial switch are not as common. However, there are case reports of ventricular arrhythmias that can occur with outflow tract–related morphologies, either related or unrelated to the surgical intervention.[28,29] ICE imaging in these patients is similar to the structurally normal heart and can be imaged from standard positions in the RA and RV (**Fig. 7**). Complications after surgical repair can include dilatation of the neoaorta, which may require imaging with varying depth levels from the RV and RA.

Ebstein Anomaly

Ebstein anomaly is a congenital malformation of the tricuspid valve, characterized by any degree of apical displacement of the septal and posterior leaflets from the atrioventricular annulus.[30] Ebstein anomaly occurs in 1% to 7% of the CHD population.[3] Left-sided Ebstein-type anomalies can be seen in up to one-quarter of patients with congenitally corrected transposition of the great arteries. Arrhythmias related to Ebstein anomaly are commonly atrioventricular reentrant tachycardias related to single or multiple accessory pathways,[31,32] atrial tachycardia, atrial flutter, or atrial fibrillation.[30] ICE is not commonly used to assess the extent of the anomaly[31] but is helpful in improving appreciation of valvular anatomy in accessory pathway ablation.[32,33] Identification of the anatomic annulus and functional annulus localizes the regions of atrialized right ventricular tissue. Catheter ablation of accessory pathways related to Ebstein anomaly is optimized from the anatomic tricuspid annulus

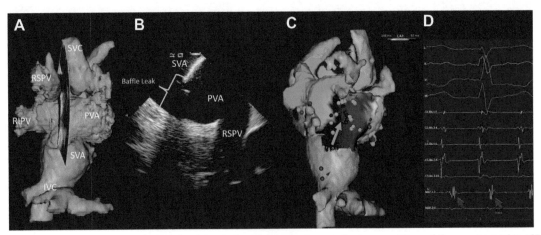

Fig. 5. MRI reconstruction with ICE of atrial switch with Mustard repair for transposition of the great arteries. ICE catheter imaging in (*A*) and (*B*) shows leak across baffle. (*C*) In the same patient, activation mapping overlaid onto MRI shows intra-atrial reentry termination site (*green arrow*) at region of baffle suture line. (*D*) Electrograms at site of termination show multicomponent signals (*red arrows*). RIPV, right inferior pulmonary veins; RSPV, right superior pulmonary veins; SVC, superior vena cava. (Images courtesy of Dr William G. Stevenson, Vanderbilt University Medical Center, TN, USA.)

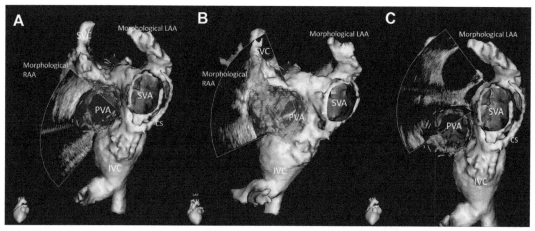

Fig. 6. ICE catheter imaging positions for delineation of PVA and SVA chambers of atrial switch with Mustard repair for transposition of the great arteries. MRI reconstruction. (*A*) ICE catheter imaging across baffle from SVA to PVA with counterclockwise rotation at the level of the CS ostium. (*B*) Further ICE catheter counterclockwise rotation with posterior deflection for imaging through the SVC and midbody of the PVA. (*C*) Advancement of the ICE catheter into the midlevel of the SVA to visualize superior anatomy. LAA, left atrial appendage. (Images courtesy of Dr William G. Stevenson, Vanderbilt University Medical Center, TN, USA.)

(TA) and not the functional annulus[34] (**Fig. 8A**). ICE can be used to visualize the cross section of the right coronary artery (RCA) from the RA. Withdrawing the ICE catheter from the middle of the RA identifies the RCA at the level of the inferior anatomic TA, rotating counterclockwise to visualize the lateral TA and clockwise the more septal TA. Imaging with ICE from the RV or from the low lateral RA with right deflection may be required to visualize all anatomic components of the TA and functional

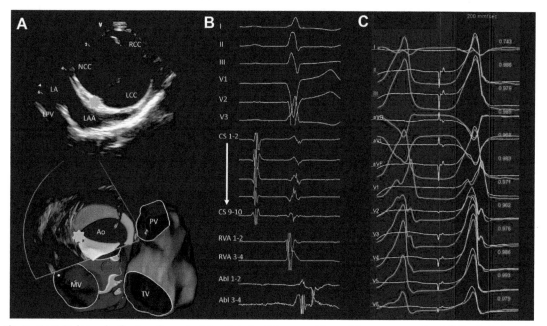

Fig. 7. Ventricular arrhythmias after arterial switch for D-transposition of the great arteries. (*A*) (*Top*) ICE imaging from the RV of the aortic valve cross section. Yellow star at site of best pace map and termination of VT. (*Bottom*) Associated imaging position on EAM in a right lateral view. Cusp reconstructions: pink, LCC, left coronary cusp; white, NCC, noncoronary cusp; blue, RCC, right coronary cusp. Yellow star at site of best pace map on the NCC side of the LCC/NCC commissure. (*C*) A 96% pace map match to clinical VT with a long stimulus to QRS duration. Abl, ablation catheter; LPV, left pulmonary veins; RVA, right ventricular apex.

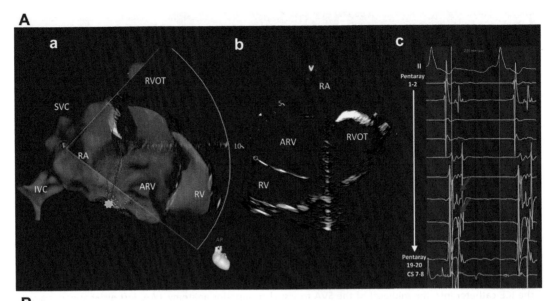

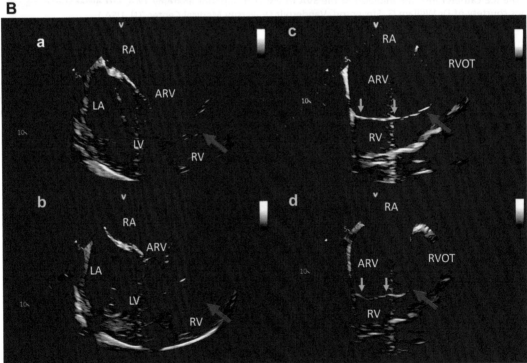

Fig. 8. (*A*) Ebstein anomaly. (*a*) EAM reconstruction of the RA, atrialized RV (ARV) and RV (*green structure*) and ICE catheter position for visualization through the TV. Red line delineates the separation of the anatomic TV from the ARV. Functional valve located at site between the ARV and RV. Successful site of ablation of an inferior TV accessory pathway. (*b*) Corresponding ICE image of RA, ARV, and RV. (*c*) Electrograms at site of successful ablation showing polarity reversal of accessory pathway potential between corresponding bipoles of mapping catheter (*red arrows*) during orthodromic atrioventricular reentrant tachycardia. (*B*) Ebstein anomaly throughout the cardiac cycle on ICE. Imaging from the low lateral RA during end diastole (*a*) and systole (*b*). Imaging from the mid-RA without ICE catheter deflection during end diastole (*c*) and systole (*d*). Red arrows are tethered points of the leaflet. Green arrow shows fixed apical displaced leaflet.

annulus. The functional level of the valve can be visualized with a standard long-axis view from the mid-RA. The degree of leaflet displacement can be interrogated with rotation from this position or by placing the catheter in the low RA with right deflection for the IVS and the extent of the septal leaflet (see **Fig. 8B**).

Bicuspid Aortic Valve

Bicuspid aortic valve (BAV) is a common congenital cardiac anomaly that can occur in 0.9% to 2% of the general population[35] and is 1.5 times more prevalent in men than in women.[1] Often BAV is seen in the presence of other congenital defects, especially aortopathies. Complications related to BAV include aortic stenosis, aortic regurgitation, and endocarditis. BAV has been shown to be a substrate for ventricular arrhythmias[36] (**Fig. 9**). Imaging with ICE in a long axis of the aorta is best performed from the RA with clockwise rotation; depending on the BAV type, this may not clearly delineate the leaflets.

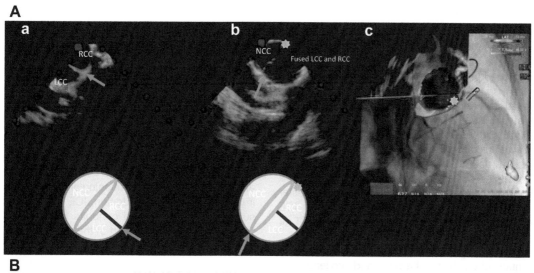

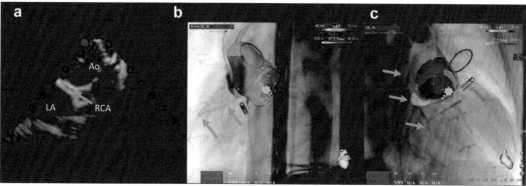

Fig. 9. (*A*) BAV with an anomalous RCA off the left main coronary artery (LMCA) ostium in an adolescent patient with premature ventricular contraction (PVC)/VT from the fused RCC. (*a*) ICE imaging of the fused RCC and LCC leaflets (*green arrow*). Lower schematic (modified from Sievers and colleagues[35]) shows a type 1 (1 raphe) of the BAV of the same ICE image. (*b*) ICE imaging with slight withdrawal of catheter to visualize BAV with the delineation of the raphe between NCC and the fused LCC and RCC (*green arrows*). Successful ablation at RCC side of the NCC/RCC commissure (*gold star*). Corresponding schematic showing a type 1 (1 raphe) of the BAV of the same ICE image. (*c*) EAM reconstruction in RAO view of the aortic activation map and ablation lesions at site of PVC/VT cessation (*gold star*) overlaid on top of aortagram. (B) BAV with an anomalous RCA off the LMCA ostium in an adolescent patient with PVC/VT from the fused RCC. (*a*) ICE image showing course of the anomalous RCA tracking posteriorly from the LMCA ostium between the anterior LA and aorta (*green arrows*). (*b*) EAM reconstruction in LAO view and (*c*) RAO view of the aortic activation map and ablation lesions at site of PVC/VT cessation (*gold star*) overlaid on top of an aortagram. Course of RCA shown by green arrows. (Images courtesy of Dr Mark Walsh, Bristol Children's Hospital, UK.)

Repositioning the ICE catheter in the RVOT and rotating until a cross section of the aorta is seen is preferred in order to clearly identify the leaflets.

DISCUSSION

Kean and colleagues[37] found that geometry definition with ICE as an adjunct to EAM for catheter ablation in the pediatric and CHD population is feasible, often useful, does not significantly prolong the procedure, and offers results comparable with standard technology. Preprocedural and intraprocedural imaging in the adult CHD cohort play an important role in successful procedures.[6] Preprocedural CT and MRI are valuable in procedure planning but require integration to the EAM systems for catheter guidance. Registration of anatomy can be challenging and has varying degrees of error related to preprocedure scan rhythm, fluid differences between scan and procedure, positional changes because of respiration, and identification of critical anatomic fiducial points for alignment. Real-time imaging of anatomy with ICE enables visualization of anatomic structures and, depending on the EAM system used, integration of ICE (Cartosound, Biosense Webster, Irwindale, CA) to generate ICE derived 3D anatomic reconstructions to register preprocedural CT or MRI anatomy. Online ICE visualization therefore is complimentary to CT or MRI preprocedure imaging.

In 18 patients with atrial switch or extracardiac Fontan circulations, Laredo and colleagues[38] showed that transbaffle/transconduit puncture could be successfully performed without echocardiographic guidance. This alternative technique used preprocedure CT and required registration to the EAM system before positioning of the ablation catheter at the preferred puncture site and then placement of the needle under fluoroscopic guidance. Time taken to puncture to the PVA was 78 minutes (range, 55–185 minutes) and overall fluoroscopy was 23 minutes (range, 7–53 minutes); however, time taken to register the CT was not reported. Time taken to image with ICE is not widely reported. Similarly, percutaneously closed ASDs have been crossed under ICE guidance when access to the LA is required to treat atrial arrhythmias.[17] Although no residual shunts were shown during follow up (14 ± 4 months), traditional assessments under TEE were not performed.[39]

There are limited data directly comparing clinical outcomes with and without use of ICE for catheter ablation in patients with CHD. In a prospective single center study of children and young adults with supraventricular tachycardia, Mah and colleagues[40] showed there were no significant differences between EAM and ICE versus EAM alone in acute success (95% EAM and ICE vs 88% EAM, $P = .43$). Mah and colleagues[40] also showed a median ICE imaging time of 10 minutes (range 1–40 minutes). Peichl and colleagues[23] analyzed the utility of ICE to guide procedures in 7 patients with atrial tachycardias after correction of complex CHD. Of these 7 patients, 4 received an atrial switch, 2 a total cavopulmonary connection, and a 1 had an atriopulmonary connection. Four patients had CTI-dependent flutter, whereas the others had IARTs and focal atrial tachycardia. During a mean follow up of 23 ± 13 months, 72% were arrhythmia free. Although access to the technology in some areas may be a limitation, a potential reduction in time and ionizing radiation exposure is valuable in this young patient group.[38]

SUMMARY

Catheter ablation of arrhythmias in CHD can be a challenging undertaking with often complicated anatomic considerations. Understanding this anatomy and the prior surgical repairs is key to procedural planning and a successful outcome. ICE adds complimentary real-time visualization of anatomy and catheter positioning along with other imaging modalities. In addition, ICE can visualize suture lines, baffles, and conduits from repaired CHD and forms a useful part of the toolkit required to deal with these complex arrhythmias.

CLINICS CARE POINTS

- ICE is complimentary to fluoroscopy during ablation for real-time assessment of ablation catheter position and to potentially minimize prolonged ionizing radiation exposure in younger patients.

- Complex anatomic reconstructions associated with repaired CHD, areas of wall thickening, inaccessible regions caused by suture lines, baffles, and conduits can all be visualized in real time with ICE.

- Both landmark and surface registration of preprocedure imaging (CT or MRI) into the EAM may be assisted and improved by ICE.

- ICE imaging positions in patients with CHD are consistent with standard imaging approaches from the RA, RV, or CS, except when atrial or ventricular reconstructed anatomy is present.

- In pediatric or small patients, imaging can be performed from the esophagus with image quality comparable with intracardiac imaging positions.

- Transbaffle/transconduit puncture may be required when access to the adjacent structure is not available or access reduces stability of the ablation catheter for achieving an acceptable ablation outcome.
- ICE guidance is safe and effective when performing a transbaffle/transconduit puncture.

REFERENCES

1. Stout KK, Daniels CJ, Aboulhosn JA, et al. 2018 AHA/ACC guideline for the management of adults with congenital heart disease: a report of the American College of Cardiology/American Heart Association Task Force on clinical practice guidelines. J Am Coll Cardiol 2019;73:e81–192.
2. Zimmerman MS, Smith AGC, Sable CA, et al. Global, regional, and national burden of congenital heart disease, 1990–2017: a systematic analysis for the Global Burden of Disease Study 2017. Lancet Child Adolesc Health 2020;4:185–200.
3. Khairy P, Van Hare GF, Balaji S, et al. PACES/HRS expert consensus statement on the recognition and management of arrhythmias in adult congenital heart disease: developed in partnership between the Pediatric and Congenital Electrophysiology Society (PACES) and the Heart Rhythm Society (HRS). Endorsed by the governing bodies of PACES, HRS, the American College of Cardiology (ACC), the American Heart Association (AHA), the European Heart Rhythm Association (EHRA), the Canadian Heart Rhythm Society (CHRS), and the International Society for Adult Congenital Heart Disease (ISACHD). Heart Rhythm 2014;11:e102–65.
4. Banchs JE, Patel P, Naccarelli GV, et al. Intracardiac echocardiography in complex cardiac catheter ablation procedures. J Interv Card Electrophysiol 2010;28:167–84.
5. Kanter RJ. Pearls for ablation in congenital heart disease. J Cardiovasc Electrophysiol 2010;21:223–30.
6. Molatta S, El Hamriti M, Bergau L, et al. Catheter ablation of atrial fibrillation in a functionally univentricular heart: a risk-adjusted interventional approach. Herzschrittmacherther Elektrophysiol 2020;31:91–4.
7. El Yaman MM, Asirvatham SJ, Kapa S, et al. Methods to access the surgically excluded cavotricuspid isthmus for complete ablation of typical atrial flutter in patients with congenital heart defects. Heart Rhythm 2009;6:949–56.
8. Barker PC. Intracardiac echocardiography in congenital heart disease. J Cardiovasc Transl Res 2009;2:19–23.
9. Packer DL, Johnson SB, Kolasa MW, et al. New generation of electro-anatomic mapping: full intracardiac ultrasound image integration. Europace 2008;10(Suppl 3):iii35–41.
10. Ren JF, Marchlinski FE. Utility of intracardiac echocardiography in left heart ablation for tachyarrhythmias. Echocardiography 2007;24:533–40.
11. Asirvatham S, Bruce CJ, Friedman PA. Advances in imaging for cardiac electrophysiology. Coron Artery Dis 2003;14:3–13.
12. Basman C, Parmar YJ, Kronzon I. Intracardiac echocardiography for structural heart and electrophysiological interventions. Curr Cardiol Rep 2017;19:102.
13. Delacretaz E, Ganz LI, Soejima K, et al. Multiple atrial macro–re-entry circuits in adults with repaired congenital heart disease: entrainment mapping combined with three-dimensional electroanatomic mapping. J Am Coll Cardiol 2001;37:1665–76.
14. Zeppenfeld K, Schalij MJ, Bartelings MM, et al. Catheter ablation of ventricular tachycardia after repair of congenital heart disease: electroanatomic identification of the critical right ventricular isthmus. Circulation 2007;116:2241–52.
15. Kalman JM, VanHare GF, Olgin JE, et al. Ablation of 'incisional' reentrant atrial tachycardia complicating surgery for congenital heart disease: use of entrainment to define a critical isthmus of conduction. Circulation 1996;93:502–12.
16. Lakkireddy D, Rangisetty U, Prasad S, et al. Intracardiac echo-guided radiofrequency catheter ablation of atrial fibrillation in patients with atrial septal defect or patent foramen ovale repair: a feasibility, safety, and efficacy study. J Cardiovasc Electrophysiol 2008;19:1137–42.
17. Santangeli P, Di Biase L, Burkhardt JD, et al. Transseptal access and atrial fibrillation ablation guided by intracardiac echocardiography in patients with atrial septal closure devices. Heart Rhythm 2011;8:1669–75.
18. Wu MH, Lu CW, Chen HC, et al. Arrhythmic burdens in patients with tetralogy of Fallot: a national database study. Heart Rhythm 2015;12:604–9.
19. Björk VO, Olin CL, Bjarke BB, et al. Right atrial-right ventricular anastomosis for correction of tricuspid atresia. J Thorac Cardiovasc Surg 1979;77:452–8.
20. Kreutzer GO, Vargas FJ, Schlichter AJ, et al. Atriopulmonary anastomosis. J Thorac Cardiovasc Surg 1982;83:427–36.
21. de Leval MR, Kilner P, Gewillig M, et al. Total cavopulmonary connection: a logical alternative to atriopulmonary connection for complex Fontan operations. J Thorac Cardiovasc Surg 1988;96:682–95.
22. Marcelletti C, Como A, Giannico S, et al. Inferior vena cava-pulmonary artery extracardiac conduit. J Thorac Cardiovasc Surg 1990;100:228–32.
23. Peichl P, Kautzner J, Gebauer R. Ablation of atrial tachycardias after correction of complex congenital

heart diseases: utility of intracardiac echocardiography. Europace 2009;11:48–53.

24. Calkins H, Kuck KH, Cappato R, et al. 2012 HRS/EHRA/ECAS Expert Consensus Statement on Catheter and Surgical Ablation of Atrial Fibrillation: recommendations for patient selection, procedural techniques, patient management and follow-up, definitions, endpoints, and research trial design. Europace 2012;14:528–606.

25. Martins P, Castela E. Transposition of the great arteries. Orphanet J Rare Dis 2008;3:27.

26. Konstantinov IE, Alexi-Meskishvili VV, Williams WG, et al. Atrial switch operation: past, present, and future. Ann Thorac Surg 2004;77:2250–8.

27. De Pasquale G, Bonassin Tempesta F, Lopes BS, et al. High prevalence of baffle leaks in adults after atrial switch operations for transposition of the great arteries. Eur Heart J Cardiovasc Imaging 2017;18: 531–5.

28. Maury P, Hascoet S, Mondoly P, et al, French Reflection Group for Congenital/Pediatric E. Monomorphic sustained ventricular tachycardia late after arterial switch for d-transposition of the great arteries: ablation in the sinus of valsalva. Can J Cardiol 2013;29: 1741 e13–5.

29. Bhaskaran A, Campbell T, Trivic I, et al. Left ventricular outflow tract ventricular tachycardia late post-arterial switch for D-transposition of the great arteries. JACC Clin Electrophysiol 2019;5:1096–7.

30. Paranon S, Acar P. Ebstein's anomaly of the tricuspid valve: from fetus to adult: congenital heart disease. Heart 2008;94:237–43.

31. Dauphin C, Chalard A, Lusson JR. Intracardiac echocardiography of Ebstein's anomaly. Echocardiography 2014;31:E232–3.

32. Vukmirovic M, Peichl P, Kautzner J. Catheter ablation of multiple accessory pathways in Ebstein anomaly guided by intracardiac echocardiography. Europace 2016;18:339.

33. Cismaru G, Muresan L, Rosu R, et al. Intracardiac echocardiography to guide catheter ablation of an accessory pathway in Ebstein's anomaly. A case report. Med Ultrason 2018;20:250–3.

34. Cappato R, Schluter M, Weiss C, et al. Radiofrequency current catheter ablation of accessory atrioventricular pathways in Ebstein's anomaly. Circulation 1996;94:376–83.

35. Sievers HH, Schmidtke C. A classification system for the bicuspid aortic valve from 304 surgical specimens. J Thorac Cardiovasc Surg 2007;133: 1226–33.

36. Kumar S, Stevenson WG, Tedrow UB. Bicuspid aortic valve supporting supravalvular "substrate" for multiple ventricular tachycardias. Heartrhythm Case Rep 2017;3:155–8.

37. Kean AC, Gelehrter SK, Shetty I, et al. Experience with CartoSound for arrhythmia ablation in pediatric and congenital heart disease patients. J Interv Card Electrophysiol 2010;29:139–45.

38. Laredo M, Waldmann V, Soulat G, et al. Transbaffle/transconduit puncture using a simple CARTO-guided approach without echocardiography in patients with congenital heart disease. J Cardiovasc Electrophysiol 2020 Aug;31(8):2049–60. https://doi.org/10.1111/jce.14590.

39. Katritsis DG. Transseptal puncture through atrial septal closure devices. Heart Rhythm 2011;8: 1676–7.

40. Mah DY, Miyake CY, Sherwin ED, et al. The use of an integrated electroanatomic mapping system and intracardiac echocardiography to reduce radiation exposure in children and young adults undergoing ablation of supraventricular tachycardia. Europace 2014;16:277–83.

Prevention and Early Recognition of Complications During Catheter Ablation by Intracardiac Echocardiography

Mahesh Balakrishnan, MBBS[a], Mathew D. Hutchinson, MD[b],*

KEYWORDS

• Intracardiac echocardiography • Catheter ablation • Intracardiac thrombus • Pericardial effusion

KEY POINTS

• Intracardiac echocardiography provides real-time, nonfluoroscopic imaging that allows rapid characterization of anatomic variants, which limit excessive or ineffective catheter ablation.
• Early complications, such as intracardiac thrombus or pericardial effusion, are detected in the asymptomatic state with ICE allowing the operator to intervene early and to minimize associated morbidity.
• Intraoperative hypotension has multiple potential causes that require specific interventions. ICE can rapidly identify the cause of hypotension, thereby allowing the operator to choose the most appropriate intervention.

 Video content accompanies this article at http://www.cardiacep.theclinics.com.

INTRODUCTION

When used effectively, intracardiac echocardiography (ICE) provides a powerful real-time imaging platform to facilitate catheter ablation procedures. It allows rapid illustration of patient anatomy and its variants, characterization of arrhythmia substrate, visualization of catheter positioning and contact, qualitative assessment of ablation lesions, and monitoring for procedure complications. ICE technology has evolved from the original radial system to more versatile phased-array transducers. The phased-array systems have integrated color and spectral Doppler capabilities that enhance physiologic data. They also provide catheter-based deflection capabilities that allow navigation into and within chambers of interest.

Despite cautious optimism that advancements in ablation technologies would enhance procedural safety, registry-based cohorts have suggested that complication rates remain stable over time.[1] Although such factors as operator experience contribute to such trends systematically, many complications occur sporadically. Although it is impossible to avoid complications in practice, their early recognition and management may substantially decrease associated morbidity and mortality. This review discusses the use of ICE in the prevention, diagnosis, and management of ablation-related complications.

a Division of Cardiovascular Medicine, University of Arizona College of Medicine Tucson, Tucson, AZ, USA;
b Division of Cardiovascular Medicine, University of Arizona College of Medicine Tucson, 1501 North Campbell Avenue, 4142B, Tucson, AZ 85724, USA
* Corresponding author.
E-mail address: MathewHutchinson@shc.arizona.edu

Card Electrophysiol Clin 13 (2021) 357–364
https://doi.org/10.1016/j.ccep.2021.03.002
1877-9182/21/© 2021 Elsevier Inc. All rights reserved.

DISCUSSION
Using Intracardiac Echocardiography to Prevent Complications

ICE provides rich anatomic detail to guide ablation cases. Using ICE allows the operator to tailor the mapping and ablation approach to the specific patient's anatomy, thereby avoiding unnecessary or ineffective lesion delivery, which can prolong procedure time and increase the risk of local complications.

Catheter insertion and navigation
Although the purpose of this review is to describe the favorable impact of ICE on ablation complications, it is important to highlight that the technology is inherently invasive. Thus, its use incurs the risk of vascular access-related complications. Depending on the specific ICE probe used, either a 9F or 11F catheter introducer is required. Although the ultrasound image can be used to guide the catheter without the use of fluoroscopy, whenever resistance to probe passage is encountered fluoroscopy is helpful to determine the catheter location. The phased-array probe is also fairly stiff and thus produces significant axial force; when applied against a vessel wall or cardiac chamber inadvertent perforation can occur.[2] Such events are avoided by using a few basic guiding principles: (1) only advance the ICE catheter when a clear space is visualized at the transducer origin, (2) if resistance to probe passage is felt do not advance it further, and (3) when in doubt use fluoroscopy to confirm probe position. In patients with femoral or iliac venous disease, consideration of using a longer (eg, 23 cm) introducer can facilitate catheter passage and distal transmission of catheter torque.

Atrial fibrillation ablation
Rapid characterization of pulmonary venous (PV) anatomy and variants are easily visualized with ICE using a mid-right atrial probe position. A recent study found PV stenosis after atrial fibrillation ablation in 0.8% of patients, and significant long-term morbidity was seen in these cases despite intervention.[3] PV stenosis can occur because of either excessive or inadvertent ablation within the PV. Although variant PV anatomy is uncommon, small-caliber veins are missed with mapping catheters. The combination of color and spectral Doppler imaging can readily identify such variants (Video 1). Occasionally ablation within a vein (eg, carina ablation) may be necessary to achieve PV isolation. ICE can provide rapid assessment of vein diameter and flow velocity, which may presage the development of long-term stenosis (**Fig. 1**).

Characterization of the ridge between the left PV and the left atrial appendage (LAA) is a critical component of atrial fibrillation ablation. Inadvertent ablation within the appendage may increase the risk of perforation. The integration of ICE with electroanatomic mapping provides direct visualization of the course of the ridge, and tracking of the catheter tip (**Fig. 2**).

Cavotricuspid isthmus ablation
ICE provides excellent visualization of the cavotricuspid isthmus, which allows the operator to immediately identify potential barriers to ablation. These include a prominent Eustachian proximally, and pouches in the mid-distal portion of the line. These sites are often responsible for conduction gaps after cavotricuspid isthmus ablation, and recognition of these features may allow them to be targeted specifically thereby avoiding unnecessary ablation of adjacent sites.[4] Both of these cavotricuspid isthmus variants may be difficult to approach with the ablation catheter directly, and ICE can provide insight into optimizing catheter approach using a loop (Video 2).

Ventricular ablation
For outflow tract ablation, ICE imaging is indispensable in determining the relationship between the aortic and pulmonic valve annuli. These structures are reconstructed with ICE nonfluoroscopically, providing a rich three-dimensional mapping environment without the need for preoperative tomographic imaging. Critical structures, such as the coronary ostia, are tagged as anatomic landmarks to avoid adjacent ablation (**Fig. 3**). When retrograde aortic access is used, ICE is helpful in screening for potential anatomic features that might increase the risk of catheter-related complications, such as atheroembolization (Video 3). In such cases the use of long introducers may reduce the risk of repetitive instrumentation of these regions.

Ventricular ablation of intracavitary structures is an important niche for ICE. Occasionally arrhythmias may originate from unanticipated structures, such as intracavitary trabeculations. Failure to recognize these variants may result in targeting adjacent regions and increasing the risk of ablation-related complications (**Fig. 4**).

Transseptal catheterization
Many operators use ICE primarily for transseptal catheterization. Phased-array ICE is uniquely suited for this purpose in light of its navigability and its field of view. The entire vertical dimension of the fossa is easily visualized with the catheter in a neutral right atrial position. Clockwise or counterclockwise rotation of the catheter allows the

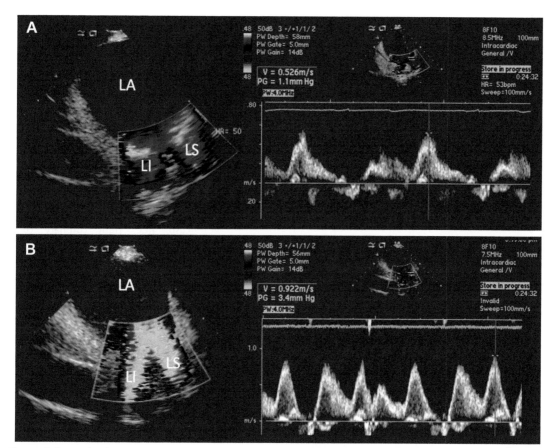

Fig. 1. Color and pulse wave Doppler images taken before (*A left, right*) and after (*B left, right*) ablation of the left pulmonary veins. Note the decrease in diameter of the left superior (LS) and left inferior (LI) veins after ablation because of edema. There is a concomitant increase in pulse Doppler flow velocity. LA, left atrium.

anterior-posterior dimension of the fossa to be viewed. In addition to visualization of the transseptal sheath-needle apparatus, ICE allows the operator to visualize far-field structures so that the angle of crossing is fine-tuned (**Fig. 5**). This is incredibly valuable for such procedures as balloon ablation or left appendage occlusion in which specific crossing locations are required. Abnormalities of the interatrial septum are rapidly diagnosed, and adjustments made to the crossing approach accordingly (**Fig. 6**). Interatrial communications, such as patent foramen ovale or atrial septal

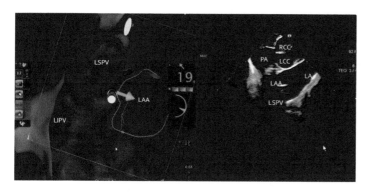

Fig. 2. (*Left*) Ablation of the ridge between the left superior pulmonary vein (LSPV) and the LAA. (*Right*) Simultaneous intracardiac echo image taken from the right ventricular outflow tract showing the ablation catheter on the pulmonary venous side of the ridge (*green marker*). Integration of intracardiac echo and electroanatomic mapping is useful in mapping and ablation of complex structures, in this case avoiding inadvertent ablation within the LAA. See text for details. LA, left atrium; LCC, left coronary cusp; LIPV, left inferior pulmonary vein; PA, pulmonary artery; RCC, right coronary cusp.

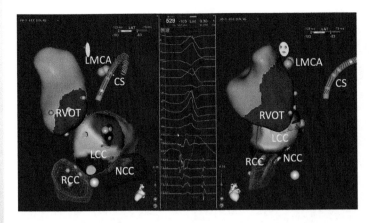

Fig. 3. Images from ablation of a premature ventricular complex from the left coronary cusp (LCC). The maps are created using integration of two-dimensional ICE slices and electroanatomic mapping. Maps are shown in left lateral (*left*) and left anterior oblique (*right*) projections. These maps can be created without fluoroscopy limiting patient and operator X-ray exposure. Critical structures, such as the left main coronary artery (LMCA), are reconstructed with ICE to avoid inadvertent injury during mapping and ablation. CS, coronary sinus; NCC, noncoronary cusp; RCC, right coronary cusp; RVOT, right ventricular outflow tract.

defect, can pose a risk of inadvertent left atrial passage and are well visualized with ICE (see **Fig. 6**). Most complications of transseptal catheterization involve inadvertent puncture of adjacent structures with the needle apparatus. Anterior punctures risk entering the noncoronary sinus of Valsalva with resulting aorta–right atrium shunt or pericardial effusion. Posterior transseptal puncture can cause perforation of the posterior LA wall. Far-field visualization of the lateral left atrial wall helps to avoid puncture with the needle apparatus, particularly in cases in which atrial septal aneurysms are present (see **Fig. 6**). The position of residual fossa ovalis in patients with atrial septal closure devices is verified, and the specific crossing approach tailored to the individual patient. ICE can demonstrate significant thickening of the fossa ovalis in patients with prior transseptal catheterization or surgical instrumentation. A

detailed survey of the fossa in these patients may identify an alternative site of crossing that is less thickened. In selected cases ICE may help inform the use of adjunctive septal crossing technologies (eg, electrocautery) in more challenging cases.

Using Intracardiac Echocardiography to Detect and Manage Complications

Intracardiac thrombus

The presence of intracardiac thrombus poses a risk of embolic complications during catheter mapping and ablation. Spontaneous thrombi may still occur in patients receiving systemic anticoagulation, and failure to diagnose them can lead to inadvertent mechanical dislodgement (Video 4). For patients undergoing atrial fibrillation ablation, ICE allows a detailed survey of the left atrium and LAA. This is easily accomplished by placing

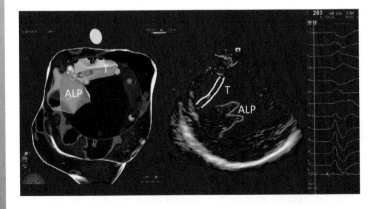

Fig. 4. The integration of ICE and electroanatomic mapping is particularly useful in the ablation of ventricular arrhythmias originating from intracavitary structures. These images are taken from a case of a patient with incessant premature ventricular complexes originating from an oblique trabeculation (T) in the left ventricle. Two-dimensional ICE slices are manually contoured (*middle panel*) and resulting three-dimensional structures displayed in the electroanatomic map (*left panel*). The representative bipolar and unipolar electrograms for the clinical premature ventricular complex (PVC) are shown in the *right panel*. ALP, anterolateral papillary muscle.

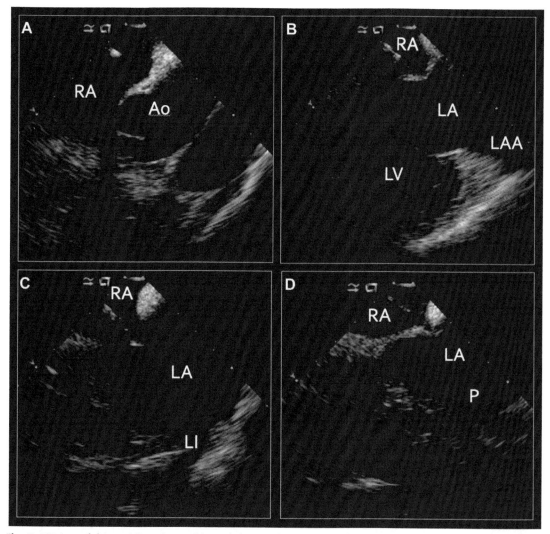

Fig. 5. ICE is useful in guiding the position of the needle apparatus during transseptal catheterization. When positioned in the mid right atrium, ICE provides near-field imaging of the fossa ovalis. The imaging sector is rotated in a clockwise or counterclockwise fashion to visualize the tip of the transseptal sheath. By examining the far-field structures for each needle position, the direction of crossing is optimized by fine-tuning the needle position. Anterior puncture incurs a risk of aortic puncture (*A*). Left ventricular access is optimized by an anterior puncture site (*B*). Visualization of the left pulmonary veins provides an optimal crossing location for left atrial ablation (*C*). Posterior transseptal punctures incur a risk of posterior wall (P) perforation (*D*). Ao, aorta; LA, left atrium; LI, left inferior pulmonary vein; RA, right atrium.

the probe in the mid-right atrium along the fossa ovalis. Although the LAA is visible in the far field with standard right atrial views, detailed imaging is severely limited in patients with LA dilation or poor acoustic windows. To definitively exclude LAA thrombus, most patients require additional views from the right ventricle (RV), proximal pulmonary artery, or distal coronary sinus (**Fig. 7**). Direct left atrial imaging can also provide excellent views of the LAA; however, this requires dedicated transseptal catheterization when a patent foramen

ovale is absent. We find that imaging from the proximal pulmonary artery is the most reproducible and convenient location of LAA imaging and is accomplished with a modest learning curve.

New thrombosis can also occur during ablation procedures and is undetectable without real-time imaging, such as ICE. These thrombi most often form on catheter introducers; however, catheter-associated clots can also occur. Occasionally these thrombi can occur during transseptal catheterization, and their recognition avoids transmitting

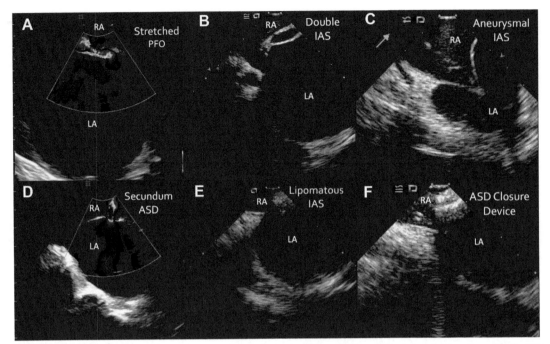

Fig. 6. ICE permits detailed characterization of morphologic abnormalities of the interatrial septum (*A–F*). ASD, atrial septal defect; IAS, interatrial septum; LA, left atrium; PFO, patent foramen ovale; RA, right atrium.

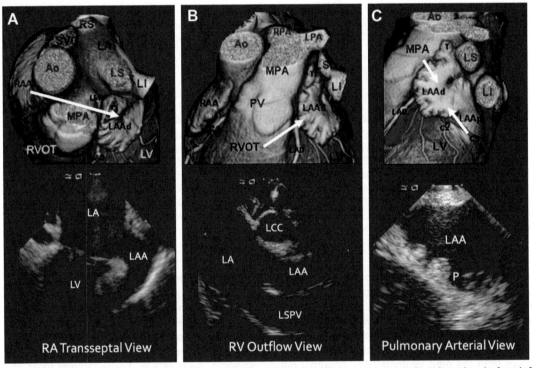

Fig. 7. Visualization of the LAA with ICE is useful to exclude the presence of intracardiac thrombus before left atrial instrumentation or cardioversion. Corresponding imaging planes with cardiac computed tomography (*upper*) and ICE (*lower*) from the right atrium (*A*), right ventricular outflow tract (*B*), and pulmonary artery (*C*) are shown. LCC, left coronary cusp; LV, left ventricle; MPA, main pulmonary artery; P, pectinate muscle; RAA, right atrial appendage; RVOT, right ventricular outflow tract; SVC, superior vena cava.

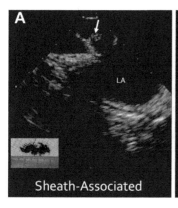
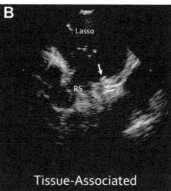

Fig. 8. Early detection of intracardiac thrombus with ICE can allow the operator to mitigate potential embolic complications. (*A*) A large thrombus (*arrow*) is seen adherent to the transseptal sheath before left atrial access. The thrombus is visualized after successful aspiration through the sheath. (*B*) A mobile thrombus (*arrow*) is seen adherent to the left atrial wall after ablation of the right superior pulmonary vein (RS). LA, left atrium.

them to the left atrium (**Fig. 8**). The administration of intravenous heparin before transseptal catheterization may decrease the risk of catheter-associated thrombus.[5] Rarely, tissue-associated thrombosis can occur after ablation because of endothelial injury (see **Fig. 8**). Specific techniques are used to manage catheter- versus sheath-associated thrombi.[6]

Pericardial effusion

Traumatic pericardial effusion is a dreaded complication of catheter ablation. It can occur with inadvertent catheter perforation during mapping or during ablation. There may be a temporal delay between the timing of the perforation and the emergence of clinical signs. ICE allows rapid screening for pericardial effusion throughout the procedure. In the absence of prior pericardiotomy, most pericardial effusions are circumferential and are seen with ICE imaging from either the right atrium or RV (Video 5). It is useful to obtain baseline imaging for effusion before cardiac instrumentation, because a traumatic effusion cannot be excluded when first documented during the procedure. Furthermore, the size and extent of the baseline effusion are documented with ICE, providing a reference for any changes seen during the procedure. In cases requiring pericardiocentesis, ICE is used to verify that the drainage sheath is contained within the pericardial space. Changes in epicardial echotexture can provide insight into the presence of pericardial thrombus. When present,

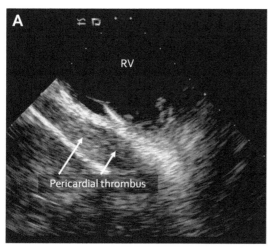
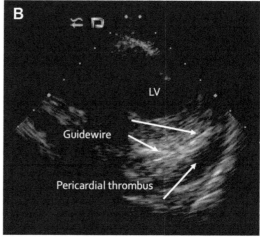

Fig. 9. ICE is useful to guide percutaneous pericardial puncture for ventricular arrhythmia ablation. Inadvertent chamber perforation can result in a pericardial effusion. Rarely, pericardial blood may coagulate producing thrombus that is not amenable to percutaneous drainage. Note the increased echointensity between the visceral and parietal pericardial layers surrounding the RV (*left*) and LV (*right*). A guidewire is seen within the posterior pericardial space.

pericardial thrombi may signify a surgical emergency because their presence may preclude percutaneous drainage (**Fig. 9**).

Management of hypotension

There are many potential causes of acute hypotension during ablation, and effective management requires an accurate diagnosis. An erroneous diagnosis leads to a delay in management and may cause inappropriate medical interventions that could worsen the patient's clinical status. ICE can provide rapid insight into the mechanism of hypotension (Video 6).

The presence of pericardial effusion is easily visualized with ICE. Left ventricular (LV) function is assessed in long axis with the ICE catheter placed in the RV. Decreased LV contractility from procedure baseline guides timely introduction of afterload reduction, ionotropic support, or the placement of percutaneous LV-assist devices. Acute volume loss or excessive peripheral vasodilation produce systolic LV cavity obliteration. Dynamic LV outflow tract obstruction can also be visualized and treated appropriately with saline administration and increased afterload.

SUMMARY

ICE is a powerful imaging tool that integrates seamlessly in the electrophysiology laboratory. The flexibility of the phased-array ICE catheter allows the operator to optimize imaging planes by navigating the catheter close to structures of interest, and its variable frequency transducer permits optimization of spatial resolution. The integration of ICE with electroanatomic mapping facilitates nonfluoroscopic geometry creation, which reduced patient and operator radiation exposure. Detailed anatomic characterization allows the operator to tailor the ablation strategy to the patient's specific anatomy, thereby limiting excessive or ineffective ablation lesions. Complications, such as intracardiac thrombus or pericardial effusion, are detected early and effectively managed using ICE, thereby minimizing their potential morbidity.

CLINICS CARE POINTS

- ICE allows nonfluoroscopic catheter navigation and geometry creation that limits operator and patient X-ray exposure.
- ICE identifies variations in pulmonary venous and cavotricuspid isthmus anatomy, allowing the operator to tailor the atrial ablation approach and to avoid excessive or ineffective ablation lesions.
- ICE facilitates transseptal catheterization by identifying atrial septal abnormalities and guiding the most appropriate location for septal crossing.
- ICE can diagnose complications, such as intracardiac thrombus or pericardial effusion in the asymptomatic state, allowing the operator to intervene effectively and minimize patient morbidity.
- The cause of intraoperative hypotension is rapidly diagnosed with ICE, thereby avoiding ineffective or potentially harmful interventions.

DISCLOSURE

The authors have nothing to disclose relevant to the topic.

SUPPLEMENTARY DATA

Supplementary data related to this article can be found online at https://doi.org/10.1016/j.ccep.2021.03.002.

REFERENCES

1. Hosseini SM, Rozen G, Saleh A, et al. Catheter ablation for cardiac arrhythmias: utilization and in-hospital complications, 2000 to 2013. JACC Clin Electrophysiol 2017;3:1240–8.
2. Pastoricchio M, Dell'Antonio A, Zecchin M, et al. An uncommon case of inferior vena cava injury during atrial fibrillation ablation. J Surg Case Rep 2020; 2020:rjaa201.
3. Schoene K, Arya A, Jahnke C, et al. Acquired pulmonary vein stenosis after radiofrequency ablation for atrial fibrillation: single-center experience in catheter interventional treatment. JACC Cardiovasc Interv 2018;11:1626–32.
4. Scaglione M, Caponi D, Di Donna P, et al. Typical atrial flutter ablation outcome: correlation with isthmus anatomy using intracardiac echo 3D reconstruction. Europace 2004;6:407–17.
5. Ren JF, Marchlinski FE, Callans DJ, et al. Increased intensity of anticoagulation may reduce risk of thrombus during atrial fibrillation ablation procedures in patients with spontaneous echo contrast. J Cardiovasc Electrophysiol 2005;16:474–7.
6. Bruce CJ, Friedman PA, Narayan O, et al. Early heparinization decreases the incidence of left atrial thrombi detected by intracardiac echocardiography during radiofrequency ablation for atrial fibrillation. J Interv Card Electr 2008;22:211–9.

Image Integration Using Intracardiac Echography and Three-dimensional Reconstruction for Mapping and Ablation of Atrial and Ventricular Arrhythmias

Alejandro Jimenez Restrepo, MD[a],*, Timm Michael Dickfeld, MD, PhD[b]

KEYWORDS

- Intracardiac echocardiography • 3D anatomy • Intraprocedural guidance • Real-time imaging
- Catheter-tissue interface • Intracavitary structures • Ablation

KEY POINTS

- Use of intracardiac echocardiography (ICE) to better understand cardiac anatomy and guide various catheter ablation procedures.
- Understand the basis for integration between ICE imaging and mapping systems with or without preprocedural imaging.
- Learn the procedural steps for using ICE-generated cardiac anatomy in a clinical environment.
- Characterization of different arrhythmia substrates using ICE imaging.
- Evaluation of tissue response to ablation therapy using ICE.

 Video content accompanies this article at http://www.cardiacep.theclinics.com.

INTRODUCTION

Intracardiac echocardiography (ICE) has transformed the way cardiac electrophysiologists approach arrhythmias by improving their understanding of the cardiac anatomy and the relevant intracardiac structures where many atrial and ventricular arrhythmias (VAs) originate. Besides fluoroscopy (with its limited ability to visualize intracardiac structures and poor spatial resolution), ICE remains the only clinically available imaging modality for real-time imaging of cardiac structures during electrophysiology (EP) ablation procedures. Compared with other modalities with potential for real-time procedural guidance, such as cardiac magnetic resonance (MR) and cardiac computed tomography (CT) imaging, incorporating ICE in the EP laboratory does not require remodeling of the physical workspace to accommodate a large gantry (cardiac CT and MR imaging), or redesigning essential EP equipment to safely perform procedures in an MR imaging environment.

This article reviews the basis for ICE-generated three-dimensional (3D) anatomy and integration with 3D mapping systems and other cardiac imaging modalities to enhance anatomic understanding and improve guidance for complex ablations of atrial and VAs. It provides clinical examples of representative

[a] Section of Cardiology, Marshfield Clinic Health System, 1000 North Oak Avenue, Marshfield, WI 54449, USA;
[b] Section of Cardiac Electrophysiology, Maryland Arrhythmia and Cardiac Imaging Group (MACIG), University of Maryland School of Medicine, 22 South Greene Street, Room N3W77, Baltimore, MD 21201, USA
* Corresponding author.
E-mail address: jimenezrestrepo.alejandro@marshfieldclinic.org

Card Electrophysiol Clin 13 (2021) 365–380
https://doi.org/10.1016/j.ccep.2021.03.007
1877-9182/21/© 2021 Elsevier Inc. All rights reserved.

arrhythmia cases where the use of this technology is key to a safe and successful outcome.

PRINCIPLES OF IMAGE INTEGRATION

The purpose of image integration is to combine the characteristics of 2 separate and complementary imaging modalities, and to integrate them into a single, clinically useful image dataset that provides key anatomic and electrophysiologic information to help guide ablation procedures. The integration between ICE, 3D electroanatomic mapping (3DEAM) systems, and other image modalities follows several basic steps, achieved manually (when using preoperative image integration) or using automated software (as with ICE/3DEAM integrated systems). These steps include coregistration using anatomic landmarks common to both image datasets (fiducial pairs), image alignment, scaling, calibration, and/or rotation. The fused image is then used in the EP laboratory to guide the ablation procedure[1] (**Figure 1**B).

With manual registration, clinicians should expect registration errors in the range of 1 to 3 mm, between 3DEAM and preprocedural CT and MR imaging studies.[2–6] Several factors may affect intraprocedural accuracy and coregistration. When using preoperative imaging, the patients' intravascular volumes at the time of acquiring the radiologic study may differ from those at the beginning of the procedure, thus leading to volumetric differences in the cardiac chambers between the 2 datasets. In addition, increases in intravascular volume during the procedure can lead to thoracic impedance changes that cause distortion of the 3DEAM geometry. Another factor is metallic distortion of the 3DEAM field by EP laboratory equipment, which can lead to inaccuracies with location point acquisition.[7] In addition, patient movement during the EP procedure can affect spatial accuracy. Because mapping systems rely on the creation of a matrix within a magnetic field, a current flow between chest and back electrodes, or a combination of both, any shift in the patient's body position during the procedure will significantly influence the accuracy of location points, catheter visualization, and cardiac geometry.

INTRACARDIAC ECHOCARDIOGRAPHY THREE-DIMENSIONAL ANATOMY RECONSTRUCTION AND IMAGE INTEGRATION WITH THREE-DIMENSIONAL ELECTROANATOMIC MAPPING SYSTEMS AND PREPROCEDURAL RADIOLOGIC IMAGING

The ability to generate 3D anatomy from real-time ICE images and integrate them with 3D mapping

systems and preprocedural imaging improves understanding of the complex intracardiac anatomy required to treat VAs, left-sided atrial arrhythmias, and arrhythmias in patients with acquired and congenital structural heart disease. Quantitative and qualitative analysis of the tissue characteristics under ICE provides valuable information on arrhythmia substrate and tissue response to ablation. Many electrophysiologists have limited training in understanding and acquiring echocardiographic images, by virtue of limited exposure during training, availability of the technology in their region/country, costs of the technology, or a combination of these. By incorporating ICE 3D reconstructed anatomy within the more familiar 3D mapping imaging environment, even operators with less experience with ICE image acquisition can easily understand and correlate the structures visualized on ICE with the anatomic regions of interest and the 3DEAM data to help them understand the origin and mechanism of a patient's arrhythmia.

The only commercially available mapping system that has an integrated module for real-time 3D reconstruction and fusion of ICE images in a 3DEAM environment is Carto (Biosense Webster, Diamond Bar, CA). The CartoSOUND module uses a vendor-specific ICE catheter with an integrated magnetic sensor, visualized in the system's 3D magnetic field. With catheter manipulation, the operator can acquire multiple two-dimensional (2D) slices of a specific chamber or structure. Once enough slices are acquired, the borders of a given structure can be segmented or delineated and the combination of these stacked 2D segmented images creates a 3D volumetric representation of the region of interest (**Fig. 2** and video 1). ICE-based geometry is also gated to the patient's electrocardiogram (ECG) and each slice is acquired in the same phase of the cardiac cycle. The integration of ICE-generated anatomy with voltage, isochronal, activation, or propagation maps is then used to guide the ablation procedure. In addition, the real-time ICE images provide additional information that may determine a successful procedural outcome, such as tissue characteristics, catheter-to-tissue contact, catheter stability, local tissue response to catheter energy delivery (edema formation), and real-time monitoring for potential complications (such as steam pops or cardiac perforations with tamponade).

Creation of multiple 3D ICE-based maps allows the delineation of separate endocavitary structures such as the papillary muscles, moderator band, aortic cusps, dense scar regions, pulmonary veins (PVs), and the left atrial appendage. In addition, maps of relevant epicardial and extracardiac structures can also be used to safely guide ablation

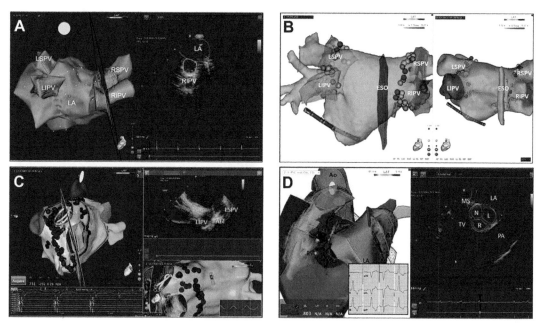

Fig. 1. ICE-generated geometry for integration with 3DEAM systems and preprocedural imaging. (*Panel A, left*) ICE-generated geometry of the left atrium (LA) and pulmonary veins (PVs) using the CartoSOUND module. (*Panel A, right*) A cross-sectional view of the ICE field of view shows a short axis of the LA and right inferior PV (RIPV) with manual border annotation of each structure. (*Panel B, left*) CartoSOUND-generated geometry of the esophagus (ESO; *ochre*) and PV ostia (*gray*) merged with preprocedural CT anatomy (*blue*) during PV isolation procedure. Ablation lesions annotated directly on the merged image (*red and pink tags*). (*Panel B, right*) Fast anatomic mapping (FAM)–generated geometry of the LA, PV, and ESO of the same patient. Note the correlation accuracy of both image datasets. (*Panel C, left*) Merged CartoSOUND and FAM geometry of the LA and PV in left posterior oblique view during PVI. Ablation catheter (Abl) is positioned in the left carina and lasso catheter in the left superior PV (LSPV). (*Panel C, right bottom*) Corresponding ICE field of view during ablation. (*Panel C, right top*) Posterior view of the ICE/FAM map. (*Panel D, left*) CartoSOUND anatomic reconstruction of the right ventricle (RV) and right ventricular outflow tract (RVOT), pulmonary artery (PA), aorta (Ao), and LA for ablation of ventricular premature beats (VPBs) (*insert*) originating from the posteroseptal aspect of the RVOT. The activation map of the RVOT during VPBs is fused with the ICE-generated geometry to guide ablation. (*Panel D, right*) Cross-sectional view of the ICE field of view highlighting the anatomic relation and orientation of both outflow tracts. In this long-axis view of the RVOT, the right coronary cusp (R) faces the posterior RVOT, the left coronary cusp is adjacent to the LA, and the noncoronary cusp is adjacent to the interatrial septum at the membranous septum (MS) region. LIPV, left inferior PV; RIPV, right inferior PV; RSPV, right superior PV.

(examples include the esophagus during atrial fibrillation [AF] ablation and the coronary artery ostia during left-sided outflow tract ablations). In the same fashion, preprocedural imaging such as cardiac CT, MR imaging, PET, or single-photon emission computed tomography (SPECT) can be merged with the 3DEAM/ICE maps to add information regarding anatomy, tissue substrate, metabolic activity, and innervation.[2,8–11] In addition to the ICE-generated 3D geometry, real-time 2D ICE images within the Carto module can be visualized as a separate window adjacent to the 3DEAM window, as a slice cutting plane within the 3DEAM window (known as fan view), or both (see **Figs. 1** and **2**, **Figs. 3–9**).

Several factors may lead to inaccuracies of ICE-based anatomic maps. Because the ICE-generated geometry is ECG gated, compared with the FAM (fast anatomic mapping), where geometry acquisition is not ECG gated, discrepancies in map volume may be seen when these two techniques are combined, with FAM tending to overestimate geometry, especially when respiratory gating is not used.[12] ICE 3D anatomic maps require either manual or semiautomatic drawing of the chamber or structure contours, which can be time consuming and may introduce human error during the tracing process. It is therefore important to ensure ICE catheter stability during visualization and acquisition of the image slices, exact delineation of the chamber and structure contours, and correct assignment of each delineated contour to the correct map or structure (see **Figs. 1, 2, 4,** and **9**). Because the specific chamber geometry of an ICE-generated map is a collection of stacked 2D slices, incorrect

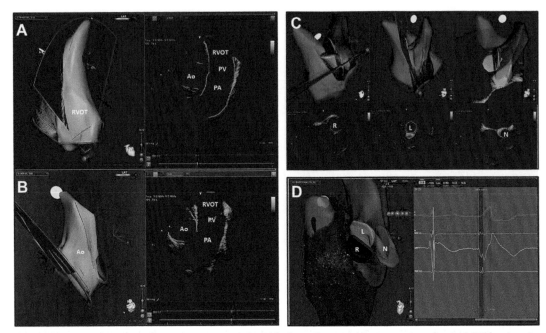

Fig. 2. Reconstruction of outflow tract anatomy for ablation of ventricular premature beats (VPBs) using CartoSOUND. (*Panel A, left*) RVOT geometry created from the combination of multiple 2D slices. (*Panel A, right*) Border segmentation on the ICE images (*green lines*) across the long axis of the RVOT and the PA. (*Panel B, left*) 3D reconstruction of the ascending aorta (Ao). (*Panel B, right*) ICE image with border segmentation of the ascending Ao (*green lines*). (*Panel C*). 3D reconstruction (*top*) and segmentation (*bottom*) on ICE images of the right coronary cusp (R), left coronary cusp (L), and noncoronary cusp (N). Note the off-axis orientation between the PA (*green*) and Ao (*purple*). (*Panel D*) Integrated CartoSOUND geometry of the aortic cusps, Ao, and PA with propagation map of the right ventricular outflow. Red area denotes earliest activation during VPB with pre-QRS unipolar electrogram at this site. See video 1.

assignment of a contour to the wrong map leads to visual distortion of the map. The correct gating during image acquisition is guaranteed as long as the ECG signal quality is free of significant interference. Problems with ECG gating or ICE catheter movement generate an image acquisition error and the system will not allow assignment of contours on the 2D slices, unless they are within the expected ECG time cycle.

Despite all these potential quality control issues, highly accurate 3D ICE anatomy merged with 3DEAM models can be obtained in a timely fashion. This article presents representative clinical cases of 3D ICE integrated guided ablation of atrial arrhythmias and VAs.

INTRACARDIAC ECHOCARDIOGRAPHY INTEGRATION IN ATRIAL FIBRILLATION ABLATION

The integration of 3D ICE images and 3DEAM for AF ablation offers important advantages, which may improve procedural outcomes and reduce complications, regardless of the catheter type and energy source used. Multiple studies have shown the feasibility and safety in clinical practice of the CartoSOUND/3DEAM integrated module to guide AF ablation procedures, with[13–15] and without preprocedural imaging.[16–18]

An important area where ICE imaging (especially when integrated with 3DEAM) has facilitated procedural advancement is in radiation exposure reduction during AF ablation. A study by Pratola and colleagues[19] evaluated 60 patients undergoing PV isolation (PVI) for symptomatic, drug-refractory AF, randomized to 3 different image integration modalities (MR imaging integration, ICE integration, or combined MR imaging and ICE integration). Although there was no difference in AF recurrence between groups at 9.1 ± 2.2 months of follow-up, both ICE integration groups (with and without MR imaging) had significantly lower fluoroscopy times (11 ± 2.3 min and 13.9 ± 4.2 min vs 23.8 ± 6.9 min, $P<.005$) and reduced left atrial dwell time (78.2 ± 29.7 min and 74.8 ± 34.3 min vs 109 ± 43 min, $P = .03$) compared with the MR imaging integration–only group.[19] A recent meta-analysis including 13 studies (2186 patients) of patients undergoing ICE-guided AF ablation (including 5 studies using CartoSOUND integration) found that use of ICE was associated with a significant reduction in fluoroscopy time (Hedges' g, -1.06;

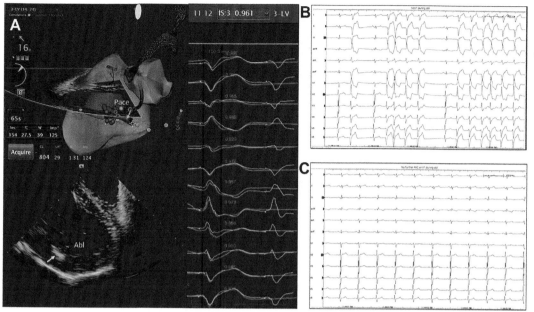

Fig. 3. Ablation of ventricular tachycardia (VT) arising from the base of the posteromedial papillary muscle (PPM) in a patient with recurrent syncope. (*Panel A, top*) FAM and CartoSOUND reconstructed geometry of the LV (*gray*) and PPM (*olive*) with ICE fan view of the LV in a transverse plane. Blue tags correspond with pace maps of greater than 96% to clinical VT and red tags correspond with ablation lesions (40 W). (*Panel A, right*) Superimposed 12-lead ECG of clinical VT (*green*) and pace map (*yellow*). (*Panel A, bottom*) Corresponding ICE frame showing Abl at the base of the PPM and tissue echobrightness below the ablation catheter in response to radiofrequency application (*yellow arrow*). (*Panel B*) Salvos on nonsustained VT during ablation. (*Panel C*) No further VT after ablation completed.

95% confidence interval [CI], −1.81 to −.032; P<.1), fluoroscopy dose (Hedges' g, −1.27; 95% CI, −1.91 to −.62;, P<.1), and procedure time (Hedges' g, −0.35; 95% CI, −0.64 to −0.05; P = .2) compared with AF ablation not guided by ICE. ICE-guided AF ablation amounted to a 6.95-minute reduction in fluoroscopy time and a 15.2-minute reduction in procedural time, without affecting procedural safety or outcomes.[20] In addition, several studies have shown the usefulness of ICE integrated with 3DEAM to facilitate elimination of intraprocedural fluoroscopy use, without compromising safety or procedural outcomes during AF ablation, commonly referred to as zero fluoroscopy ablation. Bulava and colleagues[21] evaluated the clinical outcomes of 80 patients randomized to undergo conventional PVI with or without fluoroscopy with simultaneous ICE guidance for catheter navigation. In all patients, contact force–sensing catheters and Carto 3DEAM system were used. Total procedural (92.5 ± 22.9 minutes vs 99.9 ± 15.9 minutes; P = nonsignificant [NS]) and radiofrequency (RF) ablation times (1785 ± 548 seconds vs 1755 ± 450 seconds; P = NS) were similar, as were arrhythmia-free survival and complication rates, thus supporting the safety and efficacy of a combined ICE plus 3DEAM approach, irrespective of the use of fluoroscopy.[21]

Another advantage of ICE/3DEAM integration for AF ablations is the ability to visualize and add 3D geometry of the esophagus into the 3DEAM, and to monitor for potential shifts in esophageal location during ablation procedures (see **Fig. 1**B). Unlike other strategies for esophageal visualization, such as using a dedicated mapping catheter in the esophagus or having the patient ingest contrast medium, there is no need for esophageal instrumentation or risk of contrast aspiration. Several studies showed the ability to use ICE to localize in real time the position of the esophagus and its anatomic relationship with the left atrium (LA) and PVs during ablation.[22,23] Ren and colleagues[23] published a case series of patients who underwent CartoSOUND integration with 3D esophageal reconstruction to guide RF-based AF ablation, and showed the importance of RF energy titration in areas where the 3D esophageal map was in close proximity to the PV in order to avoid thermal injury. A study by Wilson and colleagues[24] compared the esophageal locations between real-time 3D ICE integration (CartoSOUND) and preprocedural cardiac CT (1 week prior) in 20 patients

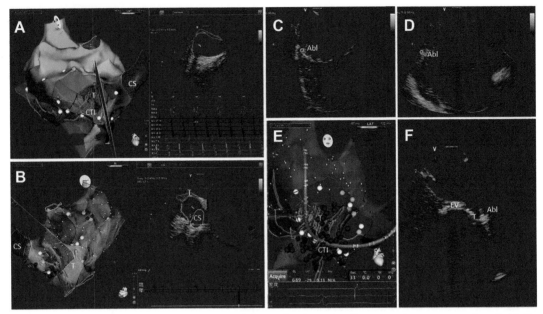

Fig. 4. Patient with prior ablation of typical atrial flutter (AFL). During first procedure, a conventional ablation was performed (fluoroscopy guided) but failed to terminate AFL. Patient was cardioverted to sinus rhythm but had AFL recurrence. (*Panel A*) Activation map (left anterior oblique [LAO] projection) of typical counterclockwise AFL (*left*). During mapping, ICE images showed a prominent trabeculation (T) extending from the Eustachian Valve (EV) across the cavotricuspid isthmus (CTI) into the right atrial septum near the coronary sinus (CS) (*right, green silhouette*). This structure was tagged on ICE (*pink geometry*) and incorporated into the 3DEAM. (*Panel B*) Posterior view of the 3DEAM (*left*) and corresponding cross-sectional view of the ICE field of view (*right*) displaying the anatomic relationship between the CS os and the trabeculation. (*Panels C,D and F*) Localization of the Abl at different positions during ablation on longitudinal ICE view of the CTI- at the CTI-tricuspid valve (TV) junction (*C*), the mid-CTI (*D*), and the edge of the trabecular extension of the EV (*F*). (*Panel E*) Final 3DEAM in shallow LAO projection with complete ablation lesion set. Extensive ablation (*red tags*) was required at the CTI and EV/trabecular extension (T) to terminate AFL and achieve bidirectional block. See video 3.

undergoing RF-based AF ablation. Overall, there was fair agreement between the esophageal locations between both modalities, but with a consistent esophagus/PV relationship in only 55% of patients. However, most notable was the dynamic location of the esophagus observed during the procedure, with 45% of patients showing substantial esophageal movement (shift in the Carto-SOUND esophageal geometry) across different LA regions.[24] Awareness of dynamic esophageal movement has important implications to reduce potential thermal injury during RF or cryo energy delivery in the LA posterior wall.

INTRACARDIAC ECHOCARDIOGRAPHY INTEGRATION IN OTHER ATRIAL ARRHYTHMIAS

Typical atrial flutter (AFL) has traditionally been a fluoroscopy-guided ablation with a high success rate in most cases (>90%); however, recurrences can occur as a consequence of incomplete bidirectional block across the cavotricuspid isthmus

(CTI). Anatomic[25,26] and clinical studies using ICE and transesophageal echocardiography[27,28] have shown significant variability in the length and anatomic characteristics of the CTI across patients. The anatomic variants that can hinder achievement of bidirectional block across the CTI include pouches or crypts, a prominent eustachian valve (EV), trabeculations, ridges, and elongated Chiari network (see **Fig. 4** and video 3). Jimenez and colleagues[27] prospectively evaluated the impact of CTI anatomy using CartoSOUND-guided ablation in 15 patients with AFL. They identified CTI anatomic variants in 8 out of 15 patients, including pouches and prominent EV, which led to an increased total ablation time to achieve bidirectional block compared with patients with smooth CTI anatomy (21.7 $\pm$ 7 minutes vs 8 $\pm$ 2.9 minutes; $P = .001$) independent of the length of the CTI (46.2 vs 48 mm; $P = $ NS). All patients with normal CTI anatómy (N = 7) had 100% catheter-to-tissue contact during ablation catheter pullback confirmed on ICE, compared with only

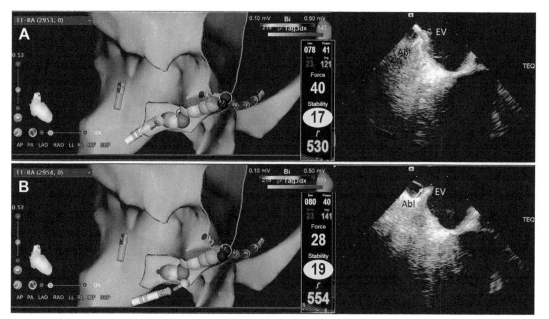

Fig. 5. Zero fluoroscopy CTI ablation for AFL using integrated CartoSOUND/FAM geometry. Patient with normal CTI anatomy (smooth endocardial surface without trabeculations). (*Panel A*) Right anterior oblique projection of 3DEAM (*left*) and ICE view of the CTI and the EV (*right*). Frame obtained during continuous radiofrequency (RF) pullback. At 78 seconds, the ablation catheter is positioned on top of the EV (*yellow arrow on ICE frame*). (*Panel B*) Same CTI pullback. At 80 seconds during ablation, the catheter falls off the EV, clearly visualized on the ICE frame (*yellow arrow*) and the 3DEAM (note the change in catheter position and contact force vector orientation). Also observe the changes in impedance (from 121 to 141 Ω) and contact force values (from 40 to 28 g). See video 4.

intermittent contact in those with abnormal CTI findings.[27] ICE-guided CTI ablation with 3DEAM integration offers the advantage of creating accurate CTI 3D geometry to help navigate the ablation catheter without the need for fluoroscopy (**Fig. 5** and video 4).

Ablation of other atrial arrhythmias where an anatomically guided approach is preferred are well suited for ICE/3DEAM integration. Examples include atrial tachycardias arising from the crista terminalis,[29] the tricuspid annulus,[30] AV nodal reentrant tachycardias,[31] and inappropriate sinus tachycardia.[32] The identification and procedural visualization of the intracardiac structures where these arrhythmias arise is key to a safe and successful ablation (**Fig. 10**; see **Fig. 8**, and video 7).

INTRACARDIAC ECHOCARDIOGRAPHY INTEGRATION IN VENTRICULAR ARRHYTHMIA ABLATIONS

The use of 3D ICE integration with 3DEAM and preprocedural imaging offers valuable information to guide ablation of VAs. The understanding of the complex intracavitary ventricular anatomy and the anatomic correlation with relevant extracardiac structures is essential for a safe and successful

procedural outcome. ICE also offers the ability to visualize endocardial, midmyocardial, and epicardial substrates, to help the operator decide on optimal ablation strategies using different approaches and techniques. Identifiable scar regions on ICE can be embedded into the 3DEAM to provide a comprehensive assessment of the arrhythmogenic tissue (see **Fig. 6**). In addition to the information provided by contact force–sensing catheters, ICE offers a unique perspective of the catheter/tissue interface. Catheter stability is greatly affected by respiratory motion, underlying cardiac rhythm, and catheter support (**Fig. 7** and video 5), all of which may influence the ablation outcome. By closely monitoring how the catheter/tissue interface responds to changes in the aforementioned parameters, ICE allows a real-time evaluation of the tissue response to ablation energy delivery (**Fig. 11** see **Figs. 3** and **7**). In addition, the ability to recognize the development of life-threatening complications such as cardiac tamponade and cardiogenic shock allows operators to provide early life-saving interventions to patients.

In scar-mediated ventricular tachycardia (VT) ablation, the integration of ICE with 3DEAM can help define the anatomic location of myocardial regions where the arrhythmia substrate resides and

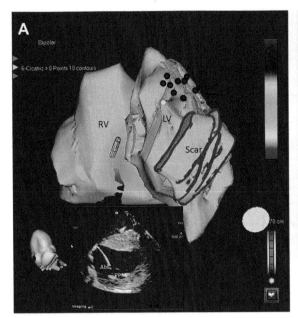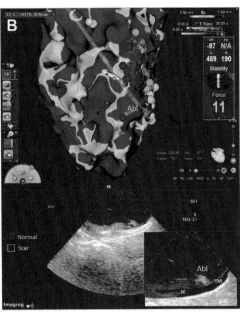

Fig. 6. ICE assessment of scar substrate in ischemic heart disease. (*Panel A*) Inferior view of ICE reconstructed geometry of the RV (incomplete and only used as visual reference), LV, and inferobasal scar (*pink*) with ICE image showing long-axis view of the LV (*insert*). Note the distribution of the scar below the PPM, making it inaccessible from an endocardial approach. (*Panel B, top*) Anterosuperior view of LV bipolar map showing extensive anteroseptal, apical, and midlateral scar. Abl is positioned in the anterolateral scar border zone. (*Panel B, bottom*) ICE view of the ablation catheter at the transition zone between the transmural (TM) and subendocardial (SE) scars.

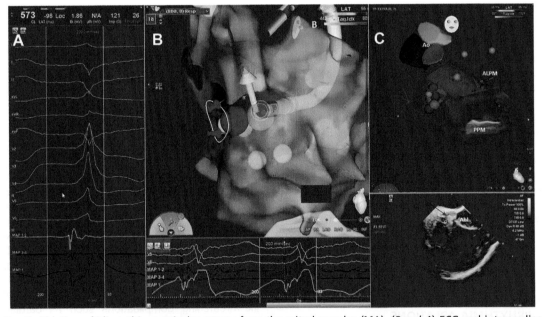

Fig. 7. Ablation of idiopathic ventricular ectopy from the mitral annulus (MA). (*Panel A*) ECG and intracardiac electrograms (EGMs) at earliest site. (*Panel B, top*) Right caudal view of merged FAM and ICE-generated left ventricular geometry with earliest activation in the posterior MA. Abl is deflected toward the posterior wall and tip is advanced into the tissue. (*Panel B, bottom*) EGMs showing run of ventricular tachycardia occurring during ablation at this site. (*Panel C, top*) ICE-generated geometry showing ablation lesions (*red and pink tags*), echo-bright area after ablation (*ochre*), aortic cusps (Ao), and papillary muscles. (*Panel C, bottom*) ICE view of catheter position and tissue contact during ablation, with echo-bright area under the catheter tip (*red arrow*). See video 5. ALPM, anterolateral papillary muscle; PPM, posteromedial papillary muscle.

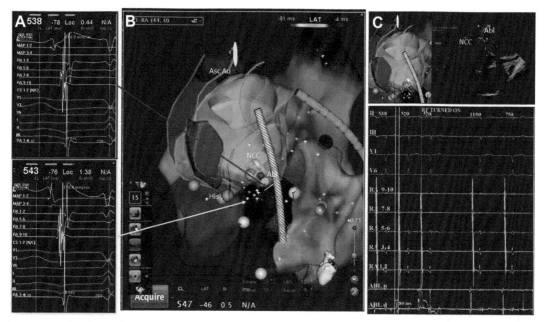

Fig. 8. Example of zero fluoroscopy noncoronary aortic cups ablation for para-Hisian incessant atrial tachycardia (AT) with cardiomyopathy. (*Panel A, top*) EGMs with earliest activation from the noncoronary cusp (NCC; *red arrow*). (*Panel A, bottom*) EGM with near-identical activation from the para-Hissian region (*yellow arrow*). (*Panel B*) Fused CartoSOUND map of the aortic cusps and aorta with FAM geometry of the RA. (*Panel C, top left*) Abl positioned at the earliest activation site in the NCC. (*Panel C, top right*) Corresponding ICE long-axis view of the aortic cusps with Abl positioned in the NCC. (*Panel C, bottom*) ECG and EGM during ablation. Within 1 second of ablation, the AT is terminated, followed by sinus rhythm. See video 7.

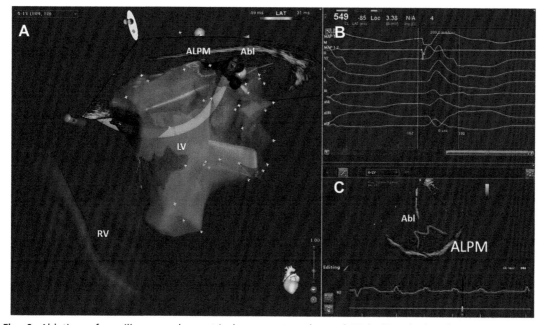

Fig. 9. Ablation of papillary muscle ventricular premature beats (VPBs). (*Panel A*) Left anterior oblique CartoSOUND-generated geometry of the RV (*ochre*) and anterolateral papillary muscle (ALPM) (*green line*) superimposed on point-by-point activation map (*semitransparent*) of the LV. The ICE fan window is projected across the LV base (cross section) to display the ALPM. (*Panel B*) ECG and intracardiac electrograms with unipolar QS signal and pre QRS activation at the Abl position. (*Panel C*) ICE frame displaying the Abl positioned on top of the ALPM (*green*) during ablation. The ECG shows a run of NSVT during RF application. See video 8.

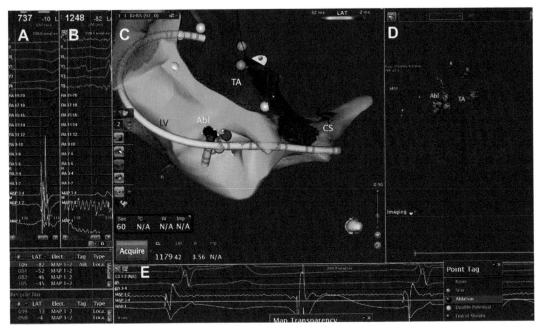

Fig. 10. Incessant ectopic atrial rhythm (AR) with paroxysmal atrial tachycardia (AT) originating from the infero-lateral aspect of the tricuspid annulus (TA). A duodecapolar catheter is positioned in the coronary sinus os, the CTI, and the lateral right atrium (RA). (*Panel A*) Earliest activation during AT (inverted P waves in inferior leads and low to high atrial activation envelope) is observed in the inferolateral TA (10 milliseconds before P wave). (*Panel B*) Activation in sinus rhythm after ablation (high to low atrial activation envelope and positive P waves in inferior leads). (*Panel C*) Activation map of the RA in right anterior oblique caudal view highlighting ablation catheter position at the successful ablation site in the lateral TA. (*Panel D*) ICE frame showing position of the abla-tion catheter and tissue contact during ablation. (*Panel E*) Earliest atrial activation during AR with unipolar QS electrogram pattern (MAP1) at successful ablation site.

guide ablation therapy. Bunch and colleagues[33] evaluated the feasibility of left ventricle (LV) scar identification by preprocedural transthoracic echocardiogram (TTE) and intraprocedural ICE, and correlated the imaging findings with scar defined by bipolar voltage using 3DEAM integra-tion in 18 patients undergoing drug-refractory VT ablation. Scar was defined using visually esti-mated wall motion assessment. The investigators found a good correlation, with 197 out of 248 (78%) segments analyzed matching scar location in all 3 modalities. However, correlation between the ICE and 3DEAM segments was superior to TTE and 3DEAM correlation, particularly in the evaluation of basal scar segments (86% vs 80%; $P = .046$).[33] A study by Hussein and colleagues[34] showed the successful integration of 3DEAM with ICE-based quantitative analysis of tissue charac-teristics and 3D scar reconstruction to define re-gions of scar and border zone in 22 patients with both ischemic and nonischemic cardiomyopathy undergoing VT ablation. Signal intensity analysis of the ICE images was able to accurately identify regions with abnormal tissue characteristics,

which correlated well with areas of low bipolar voltage on the 3DEAM corresponding with both dense scar (<0.5 mV) and border zone (0.5–1.5 mV). A signal intensity unit value greater that 137 accurately differentiated scar versus nonscar regions in all patients with defined LV scar by 3DEAM (area under the curve, 0.91; $P<.0001$).[34] A unique group of patients with inferior scar-mediated VT may present a particular challenge to ablation because of inaccessible substrate in an area below the posteromedial papillary muscle (PPM). Enriquez and colleagues[35] presented a se-ries of 10 patients with inferior LV scar and recur-rent VT who failed prior endocardial ablation. All these patients underwent a redo procedure with intraprocedural ICE substrate analysis and epicar-dial access. All patients had subendocardial hyperechoic signal below the PPM on ICE, con-firming inferior LV scar substrate, and 5 of these patients had a distinct pattern of endoepicardial scar. Despite endocardial ablation with successful endocardial electrical isolation, 4 patients remained inducible and, in those, epicardial abla-tion opposite the PPM was successful. ICE

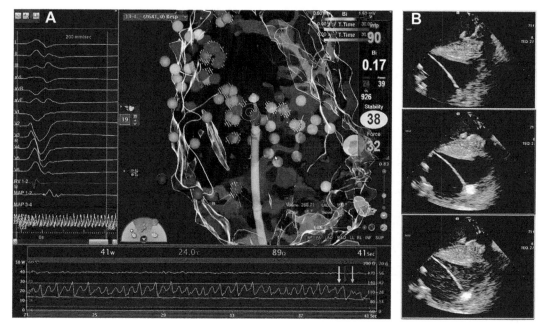

Fig. 11. Steam pop during scar modulation for ventricular tachycardia in the inferior wall of left ventricle (LV). (*Panel A, top left*) Twelve-lead electrocardiogram (ECG) and local electrograms corresponding with an area of scar in the midinferior wall of the LV (low amplitude, fractionated activity). (*Panel A, top right*) Abl positioned in the midinferior LV wall. (*Panel A, bottom*) Contact force, impedance, and power graph during ablation. (*Panel B*) Long-axis ICE view of the LV during ablation. Frames from top to bottom represent a 1-second time lapse during occurrence of steam pop. Top frame shows the catheter positioned in the midinferior wall and adequate contact with the endocardium (corresponding with the yellow arrow on the ablation graph). At 40 seconds, there was sudden development of an echo brightness below the catheter (*Middle frame*, indicated by red arrows on ICE and ablation graph) followed by an audible pop and a burst of bubbles in the LV cavity (bottom frame and green arrow on the ablation graph). Note there was no change in impedance before the steam pop occurrence. ICE images showed no pericardial effusion and the procedure was completed uneventfully. See video 2.

imaging was crucial to define the extent of the inferior scar and its intramural and epicardial extension and to guide the epicardial ablation when necessary, to achieve complete isolation of the transmural scar.[35]

In many types of idiopathic VA ablation, ICE offers unique advantages. The origin of many idiopathic VAs localizes to intracavitary structures such as the papillary muscles, moderator band, aortic cusps, mitral and tricuspid annulus, and regions where neighboring structures such as the coronary arteries or the conduction system may incur collateral injury during catheter ablation, such as the LV summit and the interventricular septum. Many case series have described the clinical characteristics, ablation strategy, and procedural outcomes of ICE-guided idiopathic VA ablations from both right ventricle (RV) and LV sites, confirming the feasibility, effectiveness, and safety of this approach[36–40](see **Figs. 3**, **7** and **9 Fig. 12**). Some centers have reported a similar outcome with ICE/3DEAM integration in a zero fluoroscopy environment for the treatment of these VAs. Rivera and colleagues[41] reported

outcomes of 26 patients undergoing ablation of LV summit VA using a zero fluoroscopy ICE/3DEAM integration with CartoSOUND. The trajectories of the left main coronary artery (LMCA) and the proximal left anterior descending (LAD) artery were traced and embedded in the 3DEAM. Ablation was conducted successfully from the distal greater cardiac vein and anterior interventricular vein (n = 9) or alternative sites (pulmonary artery = 5, left coronary cusp = 4, aortomitral continuity = 3, and endocardial LV septum = 2). Three patients had failure to suppress the VA (overall acute success rate of 84%). Most importantly, in 11 of the 26 patients, ablation could not be delivered at the earliest activation site because of catheter proximity to the LAD or LMCA as confirmed by ICE, and alternative safe sites were chosen guided by ICE/3DEAM integration. No procedural complications occurred.[41]

OTHER CONSIDERATIONS

Zero fluoroscopy ablations using 3DEAM systems are safe and feasible for the treatment of atrial

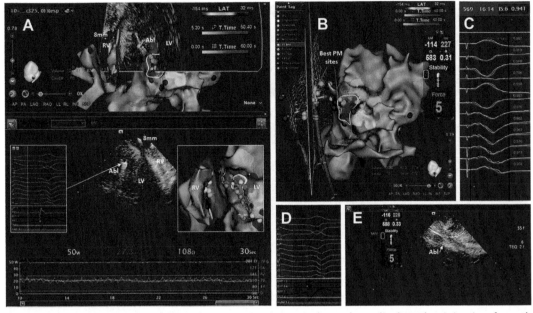

Fig. 12. Ablation of idiopathic VPBs and nonsustained ventricular tachycardia (NSVT) originating from the distal inferior aspect of the interventricular septum (IVS), after failed initial ablation from early sites in the RV and LV. (*Panel A, top*) Activation map with superimposed ICE field of view cutting across the inferoapical aspect of the IVS. After failed ablation from the earliest sites in the LV and RV, bipolar ablation is conducted with a 3.5-mm irrigated catheter on the LV side (source electrode) and an 8-mm catheter on the opposite side of the RV (ground electrode). (*Panel A, bottom*) Corresponding ICE frame with source and ground electrodes (Abl and 8 mm respectively) during ablation. Earliest local EGMs from the LV shown (*left insert*) and propagation map showing near-simultaneous early activation on both sides of the IVS. After bipolar ablation only transient suppression of PVC was achieved. Bottom graph shows power, impedance, and contact force values during ablation. (*Panel B*) Fused activation map of the LV with ICE geometry of the RV. Abl is advanced into the distal middle cardiac vein. (*Panel C*) Pace map (PM) at this site is 94%. (*Panel D*) Activation map from the distal middle cardiac vein (MCV) with unipolar QS EGM and equal precocity to earliest LV site. (*Panel E*) ICE frame of ablation catheter in the MCV before ablation (*white arrow*). Ablation at this site with half-normal saline irrigation eliminated PVCs. See video 6.

arrhythmias and VAs, and, although the use of ICE integration for 3D anatomic reconstruction is thought to enhance the safety profile of zero fluoroscopy procedures, the supporting evidence is still limited.[42] There is a learning curve required to master this technique, especially with complex ablations requiring transseptal ICE catheter access or extensive manipulation of the ICE catheter beyond the right atrium (RA). Safe manipulation of the ICE catheter in a fluoroscopy-free environment requires a thorough understanding of the cardiac anatomy, including anatomic relationships between different intracardiac structures and orientation of the cardiac chambers in the 3DEAM space. With the CartoSOUND integrated software, the catheter tip and orientation are seen in real time within the 3DEAM geometry (see **Figs. 1,3,5,7-9** and **10**). Without integration of ICE and 3DEAM, this process is more complex and requires a precise analysis of the live ICE images to ensure movements of the ICE catheter are

accomplished safely. Also, advancement of the ICE catheter through tortuous femoral and iliac veins may be difficult without fluoroscopy. Flexion, rotation, and lateral movements of the catheter may be required to advance the probe, but care must be taken to avoid transmitting excessive forward force, because vascular injury can occur. Using the Carto FAM module, geometry of the femoral and iliac veins can be obtained first with a small-caliber EP catheter to guide the advancement of the ICE probe. Alternatively, ultrasonography-guided femoral vein access and placement of a long sheath can overcome tortuous anatomy and facilitate atraumatic ICE catheter advancement into the inferior vena cava.

At present, 3D geometry acquisition using CartoSOUND is still primarily a manual process that can be time consuming. Although borders can be drawn semiautomatically, significant postprocessing is still required. Thus, the hands-on skills of an experienced mapping clinical specialist familiar with ICE visualization and the quality control from the electrophysiologist for delineating and annotating the correct structures is required for a seamless process. In order to reduce mapping time and receive the maximal clinical benefit from an integrated ICE/3DEAM map using the CartoSOUND module, the authors suggest combining 3D ICE-based reconstruction of the intracardiac structures of interest with FAM of the cardiac chambers (see **Figs. 1, 2**, **3-5**, **7-9**).

FUTURE DIRECTIONS

Because the current workflow for generating ICE cardiac geometry requires extensive operator input for the creation of multiple anatomic maps to define each key structure and operator accuracy with border delineation (manual) and correction (semiautomatic), streamlining the process using artificial intelligence applications may overcome reluctance toward its use by operators not familiar with ICE-based imaging. Pixel-based automated border detection of ICE-generated images and cardiac geometry assignment based on prespecified templates and automatic correlation with FAM anatomy could potentially automate 3D anatomy generation. Another common limitation is the need for substantial ICE catheter manipulation to visualize specific anatomic structures (for example, right-sided PVs, left atrial appendage, and cross-sectional views of the aortic cusps). Using magnet-based navigation with predefined coordinates within the 3DEAM environment, catheter movement could be automated in order to place the ICE field of view where the target cardiac structures can be visualized and annotated. The end result would be a fully automated ICE-generated 3D reconstruction of the cardiac anatomy.

Real-time 3D ICE probes not requiring 2D image segmentation to generate 3D geometry (also known as four-dimensional ICE) have been used clinically in a variety of cardiac structural interventions (including catheter ablation procedures) with early promising results, but still with limitations because of catheter size and limited field of view.[43–45]

It remains to be seen whether more vendors will incorporate ICE integration modules with their existing 3DEAM systems or those under development, but this would certainly benefit less experienced operators and those interested in lessening or removing fluoroscopic guidance for their ablation procedures. Integration of ICE-generated cardiac anatomy with ECG-based noncontact mapping technology could potentially replace the need for preprocedural imaging (CT and/or MR imaging) to define cardiac anatomy, and could result in greater accuracy with regard to localization of arrhythmias arising from intracavitary structures. In addition, as technology improves, ICE catheter size, diameter, and flexibility may be optimized without compromising image quality, allowing easier and safer image acquisition from the LA, LV, coronary sinus, and aorta. This ability could expand the clinical applications of ICE to a wider array of EP and structural procedures.

SUMMARY

ICE imaging in the EP laboratory is a well-established tool to facilitate catheter ablation and structural interventions. It allows real-time visualization of sheaths, catheter, and intracavitary structures and can safely guide transseptal access and catheter manipulation, and evaluate adequacy of contact with the target tissue for ablation. ICE 3D anatomic maps are particularly helpful in arrhythmias originating from complex intracavitary structures such as the papillary muscles, moderator band, aortic sinuses, and those arising from left atrial foci or in patients with structural abnormalities. The integration of ICE 3D images with 3DEAM is clinically feasible and provides combined anatomic and functional information to better characterize specific arrhythmia substrates. ICE is of paramount importance for early identification of potentially life-threatening complications in the EP laboratory, where early intervention can be lifesaving. In addition, as technology improves, the creation of anatomic maps will move toward a fully automated process, and, with full 3DEAM integration, could potentially replace radiograph guidance altogether.

CLINICS CARE POINTS

- ICE is the only clinically available advanced real-time imaging modality to facilitate EP procedural guidance. It is particularly useful for evaluation of intracardiac structures, arrhythmia substrate, catheter contact to tissue, tissue response to catheter ablation, and monitoring for intraprocedural complications.

- Unlike image integration between preprocedural imaging and 3DEAM, which is largely a manual process, ICE/3DEAM image integration is ECG gated and automatic, and is based on magnetic localization of ICE images within the 3D matrix of the 3DEAM system. This system produces anatomic maps of high spatial resolution with no, or minimal, registration error.

- The creation of ICE-based 3D cardiac geometry does require operator knowledge of cardiac anatomy, ultrasonography image interpretation, and segmentation process in order to provide clinically useful anatomic maps.

- The incorporation of 3D ICE geometry into 3DEAM systems is an important tool for developing a safe, fluoroscopy-free ablation environment.

- 3D ICE/3DEAM integration is particularly useful for anatomically based ablations, where intracavitary catheter navigation and tissue contact is crucial for a successful outcome. This technique is particularly important for ablation of arrhythmias originating in the papillary muscles, moderator band, aortic cusps, and other areas where anatomic variants are encountered. Neither fluoroscopy nor 3DEAM can visualize intracardiac structures to guide these ablations.

DISCLOSURE

Dr. A. Jimenez Restrepo reports research support from Catheter Precision. Dr. T.M. Dickfeld reports research support from Biosense Webster and Catheter Precision.

SUPPLEMENTARY DATA

Supplementary data related to this article can be found online at https://doi.org/10.1016/j.ccep.2021.03.007.

REFERENCES

1. Jimenez A, Dickfeld T. Computer tomography in cardiac electrophysiology. In: Zipes D, editor. Cardiac electrophysiology: from cell to bedside. 7th edition. Philadelphia, PA: Elsevier; 2017. p. 1120.
2. Dickfeld T, Tian J, Ahmad G, et al. MRI-Guided ventricular tachycardia ablation: integration of late gadolinium-enhanced 3D scar in patients with implantable cardioverter-defibrillators. Circ Arrhythm Electrophysiol 2011;4(2):172–84.
3. Itoh T, Sasaki S, Kimura M, et al. Three-dimensional cardiac image integration of electroanatomical mapping of only left atrial posterior wall with CT image to guide circumferential pulmonary vein ablation. J Interv Card Electrophysiol 2010;29(3):167–73.
4. Richmond L, Rajappan K, Voth E, et al. Validation of computed tomography image integration into the EnSite NavX mapping system to perform catheter ablation of atrial fibrillation. J Cardiovasc Electrophysiol 2008;19(8):821–7.
5. Dong J, Dickfeld T, Dalal D, et al. Initial experience in the use of integrated electroanatomic mapping with three-dimensional MR/CT images to guide catheter ablation of atrial fibrillation. J Cardiovasc Electrophysiol 2006;17(5):459–66.
6. Bourier F, Vlachos K, Lam A, et al. Three-dimensional image integration guidance for cryoballoon pulmonary vein isolation procedures. J Cardiovasc Electrophysiol 2019;30(12):2790–6.
7. Ahmad G, Hussein AA, Mesubi O, et al. Impact of fluoroscopy unit on the accuracy of a magnet-based electroanatomic mapping and navigation system: an in vitro and in vivo validation study. Pacing Clin Electrophysiol 2014;37(2):157–63.
8. Imanli H, Ume KL, Jeudy J, et al. Ventricular tachycardia (VT) substrate characteristics: Insights from Multimodality structural and functional imaging of the VT substrate using cardiac MRI scar, 123I-Meta-iodobenzylguanidine SPECT innervation, and bipolar voltage. J Nucl Med 2019;60(1):79–85.
9. Klein T, Abdulghani M, Smith M, et al. Three-dimensional 123I-meta-iodobenzylguanidine cardiac innervation maps to assess substrate and successful ablation sites for ventricular tachycardia: feasibility study for a novel paradigm of innervation imaging. Circ Arrhythm Electrophysiol 2015;8(3):583–91.
10. Tian J, Smith MF, Chinnadurai P, et al. Clinical application of PET/CT fusion imaging for three-dimensional myocardial scar and left ventricular anatomy during ventricular tachycardia ablation. J Cardiovasc Electrophysiol 2009;20(6):567–604.
11. Tian J, Jeudy J, Smith MF, et al. Three-dimensional contrast-enhanced multidetector CT for anatomic, dynamic, and perfusion characterization of abnormal myocardium to guide ventricular tachycardia ablations. Circ Arrhythm Electrophysiol 2010;3(5):496–504.
12. Khan F, Banchs JE, Skibba JB, et al. Determination of left atrium volume by fast anatomical mapping and intracardiac echocardiography. The contribution of respiratory gating. J Interv Card Electrophysiol 2015;42(2):129–34.
13. den Uijl DW, Tops LF, Tolosana JM, et al. Real-time integration of intracardiac echocardiography and multislice computed tomography to guide radiofrequency catheter ablation to guide radiofrequency catheter ablation for atrial fibrillation. Heart Rhythm 2008;5:1403–10.
14. Nakamura K, Naito S, Kaseno K, et al. Integration of intracardiac echocardiography and computed tomography during atrial fibrillation ablation: combining ultrasound contours obtained from the right atrium and ventricular outflow tract. Int J Cardiol 2017;228:677–86.

15. Kaseno K, Hisazaki K, Nakamura K, et al. The impact of the CartoSound® image directly acquired from the left atrium for integration in atrial fibrillation ablation. J Interv Card Electrophysiol 2018;53(3):301–8.

16. Nölker G, Gutleben KJ, Asbach S, et al. Intracardiac echocardiography for registration of rotational angiography-based left atrial reconstructions: a novel approach integrating two intraprocedural three-dimensional imaging techniques in atrial fibrillation ablation. Europace 2011;13(4):492–8.

17. Bhatia NL, Jahangir A, Pavlicek W, et al. Reducing Ionizing radiation associated with atrial fibrillation ablation: an ultrasound-guided approach. J Atr Fibrillation 2010;3(4):280.

18. Khaykin Y, Skanes A, Wulffhart ZA, et al. Intracardiac ECHO integration with three dimensional mapping: role in AF ablation. J Atr Fibrillation 2008;1(2):32.

19. Pratola C, Baldo E, Artale P, et al. Different image integration modalities to guide AF ablation: impact on procedural and fluoroscopy times. Pacing Clin Electrophysiol 2011;34(4):422–30.

20. Goya M, Frame D, Gache L, et al. The use of intracardiac echocardiography catheters in endocardial ablation of cardiac arrhythmia: meta-analysis of efficiency, effectiveness, and safety outcomes. J Cardiovasc Electrophysiol 2020;31(3):664–73.

21. Bulava A, Hanis J, Eisenberger M. Catheter ablation of atrial fibrillation using zero-fluoroscopy technique: a randomized trial. Pacing Clin Electrophysiol 2015; 38:797–806.

22. Kenigsberg DN, Lee BP, Grizzard JD, et al. Accuracy of intracardiac echocardiography for assessing the esophageal course along the posterior left atrium: a comparison to magnetic resonance imaging. J Cardiovasc Electrophysiol 2007;18(2):169–73.

23. Ren J, Callans DJ, Marchlinski FE, et al. 3D intracardiac echocardiography/CartoSound™ imaging of esophagus guided left atrial posterior wall ablation for atrial fibrillation. J Atr Fibrillation 2014;7(4):1184.

24. Wilson L, Brooks AG, Lau DH, et al. Real-time CartoSound imaging of the esophagus: a comparison to computed tomography. Int J Cardiol 2012;157(2): 260–2.

25. Cabrera JA, Ho SY, Sánchez-Quintana D. How anatomy can guide ablation in isthmic atrial flutter. Europace 2009;11(1):4–6.

26. Cabrera JA, Sánchez-Quintana D, Ho SY, et al. Angiographic anatomy of the inferior right atrial isthmus in patients with and without history of common atrial flutter. Circulation 1999;99(23):3017–23.

27. Jimenez A, Kuk R, Tian J, et al. Ultrasound assessment of tissue characteristics after radiofrequency ablation of the cavotricuspid isthmus in typical atrial flutter. Heart Rhythm 2011;8(5):S453.

28. Regoli F, Faletra F, Marcon S, et al. Anatomic characterization of cavotricuspid isthmus by 3D transesophageal echocardiography in patients undergoing radiofrequency ablation of typical atrial flutter. Eur Heart J Cardiovasc Imaging 2018;19(1): 84–91.

29. Morris GM, Segan L, Wong G, et al. Atrial tachycardia arising from the crista terminalis, detailed electrophysiological features and long-term ablation outcomes. JACC Clin Electrophysiol 2019;5(4): 448–58.

30. Enriquez A, Tapias C, Rodriguez D, et al. Role of intracardiac echocardiography for guiding ablation of tricuspid valve arrhythmias. Heartrhythm Case Rep 2018;4(6):209–13.

31. Luani B, Zrenner B, Basho M, et al. Zero-fluoroscopy cryothermal ablation of atrioventricular nodal re-entry tachycardia guided by endovascular and endocardial catheter visualization using intracardiac echocardiography (Ice&ICE Trial). J Cardiovasc Electrophysiol 2018;29(1):160–6.

32. Gianni C, Di Biase L, Mohanty S, et al. Catheter ablation of inappropriate sinus tachycardia. J Interv Card Electrophysiol 2016;46(1):63–9.

33. Bunch TJ, Weiss JP, Crandall BG, et al. Image integration using intracardiac ultrasound and 3D reconstruction for scar mapping and ablation of ventricular tachycardia. J Cardiovasc Electrophysiol 2010;21(6):678–84.

34. Hussein A, Jimenez A, Ahmad G, et al. Assessment of ventricular tachycardia scar substrate by intracardiac echocardiography. Pacing Clin Electrophysiol 2014;37(4):412–21.

35. Enriquez A, Briceno D, Tapias C, et al. Ischemic ventricular tachycardia from below the posteromedial papillary muscle, a particular entity: substrate characterization and challenges for catheter ablation. Heart Rhythm 2019;16(8):1174–81.

36. Santoro F, DI Biase L, Hranitzky P, et al. Ventricular tachycardia originating from the septal papillary muscle of the right ventricle: electrocardiographic and electrophysiological characteristics. J Cardiovasc Electrophysiol 2015;26(2):145–50.

37. Sadek MM, Benhayon D, Sureddi R, et al. Idiopathic ventricular arrhythmias originating from the moderator band: electrocardiographic characteristics and treatment by catheter ablation. Heart Rhythm 2015;12(1):67–75.

38. Lamberti F, Di Clemente F, Remoli R, et al. Catheter ablation of idiopathic ventricular tachycardia without the use of fluoroscopy. Int J Cardiol 2015;190:338–43.

39. Gordon JP, Liang JJ, Pathak RK, et al. Percutaneous cryoablation for papillary muscle ventricular arrhythmias after failed radiofrequency catheter ablation. J Cardiovasc Electrophysiol 2018;29(12):1654–63.

40. Proietti R, Rivera S, Dussault C, et al. Intracardiac echo-facilitated 3D electroanatomical mapping of ventricular arrhythmias from the papillary muscles:

assessing the 'fourth dimension' during ablation. Europace 2017;19(1):21–8.

41. Rivera S, Vecchio N, Ricapito P, et al. Non-fluoroscopic catheter ablation of arrhythmias with origin at the summit of the left ventricle. J Interv Card Electrophysiol 2019;56(3):279–90.

42. Yang L, Sun G, Chen X, et al. Meta-analysis of zero or near-zero fluoroscopy use during ablation of cardiac arrhythmias. Am J Cardiol 2016;118(10): 1511–8.

43. Maini B. Real-time three-dimensional intracardiac echocardiography: an early single-center experience. J Invasive Cardiol 2015;27(1):E5–12.

44. Khalili H, Patton M, Taii HA, et al. 4D volume intracardiac echocardiography for intraprocedural guidance of transcatheter left atrial appendage closure. J Atr Fibrillation 2019;12(4):2200.

45. Lee W, Griffin W, Wildes D, et al. A 10-Fr ultrasound catheter with integrated micromotor for 4-D intracardiac echocardiography. IEEE Trans Ultrason Ferroelectr Freq Control 2011;58(7):1478–91.

Electroanatomic Mapping System and Intracardiac-Echo to Guide Endomyocardial Biopsy

Marco Bergonti, MD[a,*], Michela Casella, MD, PhD[b,c],
Paolo Compagnucci, MD[b,d], Antonio Dello Russo, MD, PhD[b,d],
Claudio Tondo, MD, PhD, FESC[a,e]

KEYWORDS

- Intracardiac echocardiography • Endomyocardial biopsy • Electroanatomic mapping
- Non-ischemic cardiomyopathy • Guidelines

KEY POINTS

- The combined use of intracardiac echocardiography (ICE) and electroanatomical voltage mapping (EVM) has allowed significant increase in the diagnostic yield of endomyocardial biopsy (EMB).
- EVM enables identification of the regional distribution of disease processes, displayed as low-voltage regions in a color-coded map. This, together with the possibility of visualizing the bioptome in the electroanatomic mapping system, allows precise sampling of areas of pathologic tissue.
- ICE has an essential role during EMB, by allowing choice of the best sampling site, confirming the adequate position of the bioptome, and avoiding complications.

 Video content accompanies this article at http://www.cardiacep.theclinics.com.

INTRODUCTION

The assessment of the myocardial substrate through percutaneous endomyocardial biopsy (EMB) represents an important additional diagnostic test for cardiomyopathies of uncertain etiology. To reach a definite histologic diagnosis, it is mandatory to obtain bioptic samples from the pathologic myocardium, which can be particularly challenging due to the patchy/inhomogeneous distribution in many cardiomyopathies. In this context, electroanatomic voltage mapping (EVM) and intracardiac echocardiography (ICE) play an essential role. Indeed, when performing EMB, the accurate definition of individual cardiac anatomy and the location of pathologic substrate are fundamental to obtain adequate samples. ICE enables the operator to precisely visualize the anatomy of the cardiac chambers and to appreciate morphologic abnormalities and dyskinetic areas. EVM plays a complementary role, as it provides a functional image of the heart, picturing the diseased areas identified by low-voltage potentials in a color-coded map. This combined approach has allowed significant increase in the sensitivity and specificity of EMB, to the point that EMB is now considered the gold standard approach in specialized centers.[1–5] In this state-of-the-art review, we

Drs M. Bergonti and M. Casella contributed equally to this work.
[a] Heart Rhythm Center, Centro Cardiologico Monzino IRCCS, Milan, Italy; [b] Cardiology and Arrhythmology Clinic, University Hospital "Ospedali Riuniti", Ancona, Italy; [c] Department of Clinical, Special and Dental Sciences, Marche Polytechnic University, Ancona, Italy; [d] Department of Biomedical Sciences and Public Health, Marche Polytechnic University, Ancona, Italy; [e] Department of Clinical Sciences and Community Health, University of Milan, Milano, Italy
* Corresponding author. Centro Cardiologico Monzino, IRCCS, Via C. Parea, 4, Milano 20138, Italy.
E-mail address: bergmar21@gmail.com

cardiacEP.theclinics.com

provide guidance on how to practically perform an EVM-guided and ICE-guided EMB, and summarize the evidence supporting this approach, our final aim being to facilitate the spread of this fundamental step in the path of a patient-tailored approach to cardiomyopathies.

THE ROLE OF ENDOMYOCARDIAL BIOPSY IN 2020

The role of EMB in the diagnosis and management of patients with cardiomyopathies remains a controversial issue. The traditionally performed, fluoroscopy-guided EMB has been limited by both its low sensitivity (10%–35%)[6] and the inherent risk of complications.[7] Because of the lack of adequate sized randomized controlled studies, most guidelines usually refer to single-center registries, case series, and expert opinion. This explains the heterogeneous and sometimes discordant recommendations as provided in **Table 1**.[6,8,9]

Although technical advances have significantly improved the noninvasive tissue characterization through cardiac magnetic resonance or cardiac computer tomography, thus refining on its ability to adequately differentiate multiple cardiomyopathies, EMB still plays a crucial role in defining the underlying etiologic process. Of particular interest for electrophysiologists dealing with ventricular arrhythmias in patients with nonischemic cardiomyopathy, is the fact that a histologic analysis may display specific alterations (eg, fibro-fatty replacement, inflammatory infiltration, noncaseating granulomas) that would otherwise be missed, and may help in precisely defining the underlying pathology, thus changing the management of patients.[10–13]

HOW ELECTROPHYSIOLOGY CAME IN HELP OF ENDOMYOCARDIAL BIOPSY

The major drawback of traditional EMB is its low diagnostic yield. The low sensitivity of blinded EMB pointing at the interventricular septum is intuitive. Thus, if we really want to perform a diagnostic EMB, we need to first localize the areas of diseased myocardium, and then point our bioptome toward these areas.

The electrophysiology (EP) interest in EMB, driven by the study of patients with ventricular arrhythmias and suspected cardiomyopathies, has radically changed the technical approach to EMB, starting from 2008.[1,2]

- *EP techniques* were applied to EMB procedures:

  ○ The bioptome was introduced into a steerable sheath to increase its maneuverability in all targeted zones.
  ○ In case of left ventricular biopsy, a transseptal approach was preferred to the conventional retrograde trans-aortic approach, conferring better stability and maneuverability.
- *Diagnostic/imaging tools* commonly used in EP procedures were added: ICE and EVM.

Intracardiac Echocardiography

ICE is a unique imaging modality that provides the operator with high-resolution, real-time representations of cardiac chambers. The systematic adoption of ICE as a guide during EMB confers multiple advantages:

- A more accurate localization of the catheter/bioptome and their relationships with cardiac structures, ensuring adequate catheter-tissue *contact* (Video 1).
- A direct visualization of the sample area, so as to adequately evaluate the thickness and characteristics of the *tissue* (scar, aneurysm, bulging) (**Figs. 1–3**, Videos 2–5), which has a strong correlation with EVM.
- *Avoidance* of endo-cavitary structures (valve flaps, chordae tendineae, papillary muscles, moderator band), reducing risk of structural complications (**Fig. 4**, Video 6).
- *Rea- time monitoring* of EMB-related complications (ie, pericardial effusion, valve dysfunction, thrombus formation), so as to promptly take action.[14]
- Thanks to the lack of need for general anesthesia and second operator, ICE has nowadays substantially replaced transesophageal echocardiography.

Due to the various, previously mentioned, advantages, ICE is intuitively considered a fundamental tool when performing EMB, although no specific study has systematically addressed its efficacy when used without the EVM combined approach. Indeed, only a few published case reports can be found in the literature describing ICE-guided EMB, and they refer exclusively to biopsies of intracardiac masses.[15]

Electroanatomic Voltage Mapping

EVM allows combining cardiac electrical information and 3-dimensional (3D) spatial location information, generating a cardiac chamber 3D-reconstruction with superimposed intracardiac electrocardiogram records. This allows precise identification of areas of low-voltage or fragmented and delayed

Table 1
Level of evidence: according to different guidelines societies, level of evidence is expressed as either one of these two

Indications for Endomyocardial Biopsy According to Different Guideline Societies	
Association for European Cardiovascular Pathology and the Society for Cardiovascular Pathology, 2011	
Inflammatory cardiomyopathy (myocarditis, cardiac sarcoidosis)	S
Infiltrative diseases (amyloidosis, iron overload, glycogen storage diseases, Anderson-Fabry)	
Arrhythmogenic cardiomyopathy	
Cardiac tumors	
Heart transplantation	
Cardiotoxicity	M
Peripartum cardiomyopathy	
Hypertrophic cardiomyopathy, idiopathic restrictive cardiomyopathy, idiopathic dilated cardiomyopathy	
Laminopathies	N
Scientific Statement from American Heart Association; American College of Cardiology; European Society of Cardiology, 2007	
New-onset (<2 wk) heart failure associated with a normal-sized or dilated left ventricle	B
New-onset (2 weeks–3 months) heart failure–associated dilated left ventricle and new ventricular arrhythmias, or failure to respond to usual care	
Heart failure (>3 mo) with dilated left ventricle and ventricular arrhythmias, which does not respond to usual care	C
Suspected cardiotoxicity or restrictive disease	
Suspected cardiac tumors	
Heart failure (>3 mo) with dilated left ventricle, without ventricular arrhythmias, which does respond to usual care	C
Suspected arrhythmogenic cardiomyopathy	
Unexplained ventricular arrhythmias	
Italian Consensus Document, 2013	
No alternative method exists to reach a definite diagnosis that can have obvious consequences for clinical management	
No alternative method exists to reach a definite diagnosis; however, the implications for clinical management are uncertain	
No alternative method exists to reach a definite diagnosis; however, the diagnosis would not influence clinical management	
An alternative method exists to reach a definite diagnosis	
ARVC: evaluation of the current diagnostic criteria and differential diagnosis, 2018	
EMB is not indicated as a routine test for ARVC. It should be reserved for selected patients, such as probands with a sporadic form of ARVC and predominant LV involvement, in whom the final diagnosis depends on histologic exclusion of phenocopies, such as chronic myocarditis, sarcoidosis, and other heart muscle disorders	B
ARVC: 2019 Consensus statement on the evaluation, risk stratification and management of ARVC	
Biopsy can be particularly useful in excluding inflammatory conditions mimicking ARVC (myocarditis, sarcoidosis)	B
Myocarditis: a position statement of the ESC working group on myocardial and pericardial disease, 2012	

(continued on next page)

Table 1
(continued)

Indications for Endomyocardial Biopsy According to Different Guideline Societies	
EMB is recommended in patients with clinically suspected myocarditis	C
EMB is recommended in suspected myocarditis with life-threatening presentation	B
Myocarditis: 2013 ACCF/AHA guideline for the management of heart failure	
EMB should be performed in patients with rapidly progressive and unexplained cardiomyopathy, those in whom active myocarditis, especially giant cell myocarditis, is being considered	B
Sarcoidosis: HRS Expert Consensus Statement on the Diagnosis and Management, 2014	
In patients with extracardiac sarcoidosis, lymph node or lung biopsy is typically targeted first due to the higher diagnostic yield and lower procedural risk	B
In cases of isolated cardiac sarcoidosis or negative extracardiac biopsy, EMB may be required to confirm the diagnosis	B
Sarcoidosis: Japanese Ministry of Health and Welfare Criteria for Diagnosis of Cardiac Sarcoidosis, 2006	
Cardiac sarcoidosis is confirmed when endomyocardial biopsy specimens demonstrate noncaseating epithelioid granulomas with histologic or clinical diagnosis of extracardiac sarcoidosis	A
EMB should be recommended when noninvasive evaluation is insufficient to reach a final diagnosis	C

A: Data derived from multiple randomized clinical trials or meta-analyses.
B: Data derived from a single randomized clinical trial or large nonrandomized studies.
C: Consensus of opinion of the experts and/or small studies, retrospective studies, registries.
M: Published peer-reviewed evidence is mixed concerning the utility of the test.
N: There is no published peer-reviewed evidence assessing the utility of the test.
S: Published peer-reviewed evidence supports the utility of the test.
   Classes of recommendations are displayed as follows: Green: Evidence and/or general agreement that a given treatment or procedure is beneficial, useful, effective. Yellow: Weight of evidence/opinions favour usefulness/efficacy. Orange: usefulness/efficacy is less well established by evidence/opinion. Red: Evidence or general agreement that the given treatment or procedure is not useful/effective, and in some cases may be harmful.
   Abbreviations: ACC, American College of Cardiology; AHA, American Heart Association; ARVC, arrhythmogenic right ventricular cardiomyopathy; EMB, endomyocardial biopsy; ESC, European Society of Cardiology; HRS, Heart Rhythm Society.

potentials, which are hallmarks of diseased tissue. Intuitively, EVM used as a guide to EMB may increase EMB diagnostic yield by locating low-voltage regions corresponding to areas of pathologic substrate.[1,4,16,17] Both CARTO system (Biosense Webster, Diamond Bar, CA) and Ensite NavX (Abbott, SJM, St Paul, MN) can be used.

In addition, the bioptome, as any other catheter, can be visualized into electroanatomic mapping systems (**Fig. 5**). This enables the operator to direct the bioptome tip and to confirm its correct position, exactly where the diseased myocardium has been identified.

However, several variables inherent to the methodology should be taken into consideration when analyzing a voltage map:

- Catheter contact with tissue is paramount, as poor contact may lead to falsely reduced voltages.

- Number and density of location "points" in the map, type of rhythm being mapped, and the size of the electrodes are to be weighed.
- Both unipolar and bipolar voltage maps need to be analyzed. Unipolar EVM may yield greater sensitivity in cardiomyopathies with prevalent epicardial involvement, and spared endocardium.[3]

Intracardiac Echocardiography and Electroanatomic Voltage Mapping: a Combined Approach

Modern imaging software allows integration of real-time echographic images with electroanatomic maps. The anatomic information acquired by ICE can be combined with functional data from EVM.[18] A combined approach can be theoretically performed with all available electroanatomic mapping systems, but using the CARTO

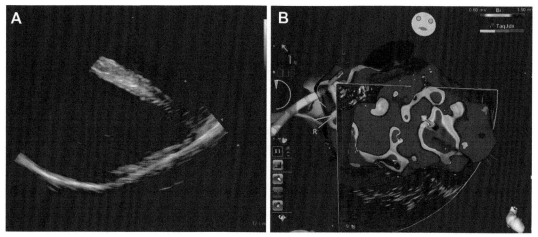

Fig. 1. Septal scar in a patient with idiopathic dilated cardiomyopathy. (*A*) Modified long-axis view of the LV. Hyperechoic myocardium in septal position is present, consistent with scar. (*B*) Merged images of intracardiac echography and electroanatomic voltage map, highlighting diseased tissue (areas colored in *red*, *green*, *yellow*, and *blue*) in septal position. Marked with the white arrow we can appreciate the mapping catheter, which is pointing at the border zone, between diseased and healthy myocardium.

Mapping System, a specific software (CARTO-SOUND, Biosense Webster), has been designed with this intent. A modified ICE catheter (Sound-Star), with a sensor on the tip, acquires ultrasound 2-dimensional slices at various imaging planes and then they are combined to obtain a 3D shell (**Fig. 6**A, B). EVM information can then be superimposed over the anatomic ICE reconstruction (**Fig. 6**C–F, Video 7).

Our Technique: a Practical Approach

Initially, the ICE probe is positioned in the right chambers to reconstruct the 3D anatomy of the right ventricle (RV) and left ventricle (LV), according to the site of interest. Operators decide whether to map RV, LV, or both based on the disease anatomic distribution, as shown by cardiac magnetic resonance (CMR) and on the presumed origin of ventricular arrhythmias. While creating the ventricular shell, areas of interest (ie, fibrosis, bulging dyskinetic segments, or thinned walls) are marked. Once the shell of the ventricle is acquired with ICE, EVM is then performed. Once the mapping phase is completed, voltage maps of the RV and/or LV are merged with the ICE-3D shell, to check for the completeness of EVM map and to assess the correlation between low-voltage areas and dyskinetic and/or fibrotic areas.

By analyzing the EVM bipolar and unipolar maps together with the ICE reconstruction, the target area for biopsy is chosen. RV endomyocardial bioptic samples are obtained through the right femoral vein via a disposable bioptome (Bipal, Biosense Webster) introduced into a steerable sheath. In case of LV EMB, the long steerable sheath is positioned at the mitral annulus by a transseptal approach.

Thanks to the steerable sheath, the operators are able to position the bioptome in correspondence to diseased myocardium. In addition to fluoroscopy, the correct position of the bioptome is usually checked through both the electroanatomic mapping and the ICE systems. We usually obtain 3 to 6 samples per procedure. Two illustrative examples are reported in **Figs. 7** and **8** and Video 8.

SUPPORTING EVIDENCE

In 2005, Corrado and colleagues[19] provided the first proof that low-voltage regions detected by EVM correspond to areas of fibro-fatty replacement in the RV in patients with arrhythmogenic RV cardiomyopathy (ARVC). Since then, 2 pivotal studies, in 2008 and 2009, described that EVM-guided EMB enhanced the diagnostic value of EMB.[1,2] A recent systematic review analyzing 17 articles and 148 patients undergoing EVM-guided EMB (144/148 in the RV, mostly using bipolar-only EVM)[16] reported the use of ICE in just 4 of 17 articles, steerable sheaths in 3, and contact-force sensors for mapping in 1. In this review, EMB sensitivity and specificity were 92% and 58%, respectively. Few studies considered the addition of unipolar voltage mapping to bipolar, as a guide to EMB.[20] When analyzing the performance of unipolar versus bipolar EVM, the former conferred slightly better area under the curve (0.81 vs 0.72, $P = .06$) and sensitivity, but the latter had higher specificity (74% vs 89%).

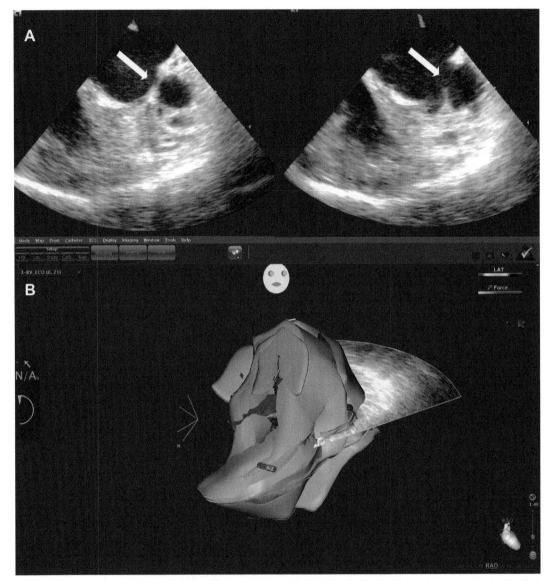

Fig. 2. Bulging of the RV free wall in a patient with RV arrhythmogenic dysplasia The upper portion (*A*) of the figure represents the apical segments of the RV, with evidence of a small aneurysm with systo-diastolic bulging (*white arrows*). In the lower portion (*B*), we can appreciate how intracardiac echographic images can be displayed into the electroanatomic map, allowing to appropriately mark thinned or aneurismal areas that are not to be sampled due to high risk of cardiac perforation.

Overall, unipolar mapping resulted in an increased diagnostic yield (63% vs 83%).[3] We recently reported on the experience accrued in our center, where 162 EMBs were performed between 2010 and 2019.[5] The sampling site was the RV in 116 (72.5%), the LV in 31 (19.4%), and both ventricles in 13 (8.1%) patients, and biopsy samples were judged appropriate for histologic analysis in 141 (87.0%) subjects.[5] Among the analyzed samples, a diagnosis was reached in 120 patients (74.1%), and EVM proved to have similar sensitivity to CMR (74%, confidence interval [CI] 66%–83%

and 77%, CI 69%–86%, respectively), with EVM having nonsignificantly higher specificity (70%, CI 56%–83% and 47%, CI 31%–64%, respectively). When both CMR and EVM were concordant, the diagnostic yield of EMB was 89%. Moreover, the pooled sensitivity of CMR and EVM was 95%.[5]

Safety

Although it is considered a safe procedure, EMB is inevitably associated with an inherent risk of complications.[7]

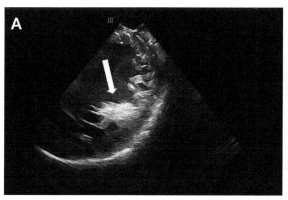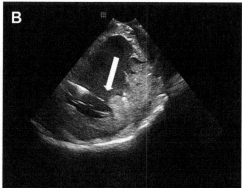

Fig. 3. Example of fibrotic papillary muscle in a patient with ventricular arrhythmias originating from the papillary muscle In the left quadrant (*A*), we can see a short-axis view of the LV from the RV, displaying, as pointed by the white arrow, a fibrotic papillary muscle that is recognized due to its hyperechoic appearance. In the right quadrant (*B*), the bioptome is visualized (*white arrow*), pointing at the base of the papillary muscle. ICE image confirms the adequate tissue-bioptome contact and the correct position.

- *Vascular access-related complications* are the most frequent (1%–3%) and usually the less dangerous. They encompass access site hematoma, arterio-venous fistula, and accidental puncture of the femoral artery. The use of ICE and EVM may potentially increase risk of these complications, due to the increased number and larger caliper of access sites needed.
- *Structural complications*, invariably linked to bioptome manipulation and tissue sampling, are instead the most worrisome, and large registers have reported an incidence rate ranging from 1.0% to 1.6%.[7] They can be divided into electrical complications or mechanical complications.
  - *Electrical*: The interventricular septum comprehends the conduction system with the His, right, and left bundles. Indeed, there have been reports of transient or permanent atrioventricular block or bundle branch block secondary to damage to the conduction system (see **Fig. 6**).
  - *Mechanical:* These may be the result of damage to specific cardiac structures (ie, papillary muscles, chordae tendineae, and valve leaflet) or cardiac perforation (0.27% of cases).[7] ICE plays a major role in avoiding mechanical complications thanks to the precise visualization of cardiac anatomy and the identification of pathologically thinned myocardial areas (see **Fig. 2**). In addition, ICE helps in the differential diagnosis of sudden hypotension: indeed, thanks to its ability to readily visualize pericardial effusion, when the latter is absent, one may consider other possibilities (eg, cardiogenic shock due to coronary artery damage, air embolism after transseptal puncture, or mere autonomic reflexes).

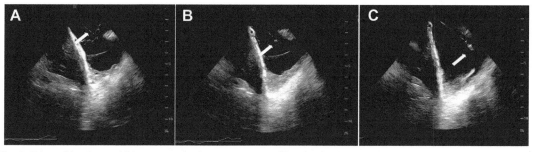

Fig. 4. Tricuspid valve and bioptome. The bioptome is a stiff catheter that may damage the tricuspid valve while crossing the atrioventricular junction. ICE enables the operator to clearly visualize the bioptome and its relation with the valve, thus allowing to reduce such complication. (*A*) The bioptome in proximity with the valve leaflets. In (*B*), the tricuspid valve is open and the bioptome is gently pushed ahead to the apical portion of the RV free wall in (*C*). White arrows points at the bioptome.

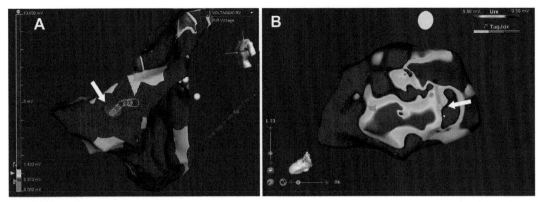

Fig. 5. Bioptome visualization in mapping systems. We see in (*A*) the 3D electroanatomic reconstruction of the RV with NavX system. As depicted by the white arrow, we can appreciate the bioptome pointing at the interventricular septum. (*B*) The 3D electroanatomic reconstruction of the LV with CARTO system. The bioptome is indicated by the white arrow.

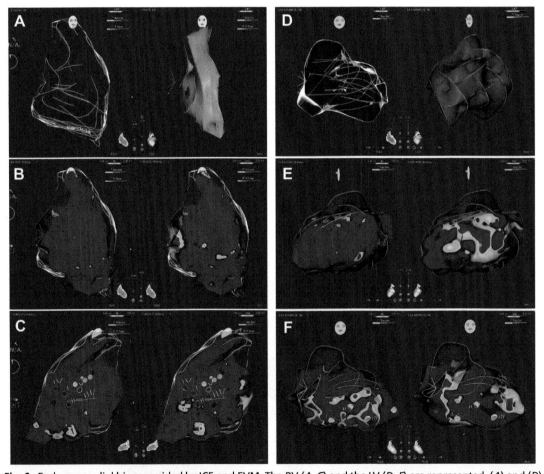

Fig. 6. Endomyocardial biopsy guided by ICE and EVM. The RV (*A–C*) and the LV (*D–F*) are represented. (*A*) and (*D*) show the SoundStar catheter acquiring 2D slices at various imaging planes, thus reconstructing the ventricular geometry. Thereafter, voltage mapping is performed (*B* and *E*), and diseased areas are superimposed in a color-coded fashion over the 3D shell. In this case, small patchy areas of disease tissue can be identified in the septal segments of the RV (*C*). As for the LV, diseased tissue is evident in the mid-apical septal portion and in the mid-lateral segment (*F*). Marked with dark gray dots (for the RV) and light gray dots (for the LV), we can see areas of myocardium that underwent sampling. Of note, while sampling the RV septum, special attention must be paid to the close proximity with the His conduction system, marked with orange dots.

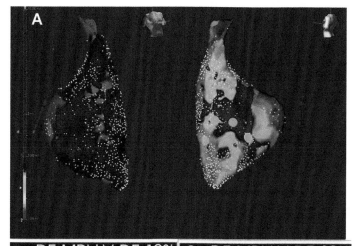

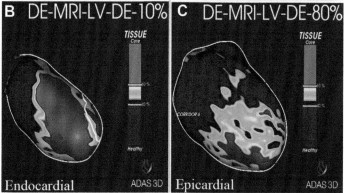

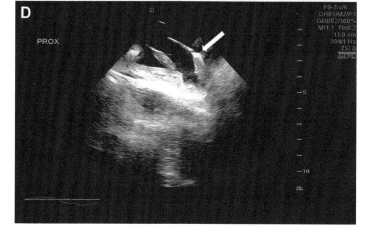

Fig. 7. ICE and EVM-guided EMB in a patient with amyloidosis. (*A*) Electroanatomic reconstruction of the RV chamber with NavX system. Purple areas represent healthy tissue. Low-voltage areas are evident at septum and anterior wall in their apical segments. Green dots show areas that underwent sampling. (*B, C*) Further information can be acquired thanks to CMR. ADAS 3D software (Galgo Medical), identifies fibrotic substrates at CMR and shows their endocardial or epicardial distribution, depicted as electroanatomic voltage map. In this case, LV GALCO images show a large endocardial (*B*) fibrosis and a more limited epicardial (*C*) fibrosis at interventricular septum in its distal segment. (*D*) The classic appearance of cardiac amyloidosis at intracardiac-echo, with evidence of thickened bright myocardium. As pointed by the white arrow, the bioptome with adequate contact with the tissue, pointing at areas of pathologic substrate previously identified is also displayed.

Specific studies prospectively addressing the complication rate with and without EVM and ICE when performing EMB are currently lacking.

Recently, 2 studies demonstrated that in patients undergoing endocardial ventricular arrhythmias ablation, the concomitant performance of EMB was not associated with an increased risk of intracardiac complication.[21,22] Thus, in patients referred for ventricular arrhythmia ablation with underling cardiomyopathy of unknown origin, it may be reasonable to complete the procedure with an EMB. Obviously, sampling must be performed in areas different from the site of current or prior ablation.

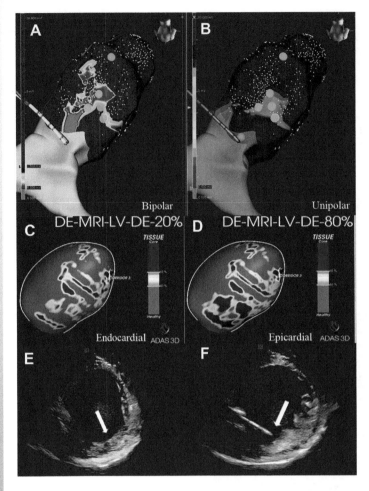

Bipolar

DE-MRI-LV-DE-20%   DE-MRI-LV-DE-80%

Unipolar

Endocardial ADAS 3D   Epicardial ADAS 3D

Fig. 8. A patient with nonischemic inferior scar. (*A, B*) Bipolar and unipolar EVM with NavX system. Inferior scar is detected and samples (*green dots*) are taken from that site. (*C, D*) CMR analysis with ADAS 3D software (Galgo Medical) confirms this finding with evidence of a large inferior epicardial scar with little endocardial involvement. (*E*) Direct visualization with intracardiac echocardiography (short-axis view) of the inferior epicardial scar (bright tissue pointed by *white arrow*). (*F*) The bioptome pointing at the diseased area so to minimize the risk of sampling error.

SUMMARY

Endomyocardial biopsy plays an increasingly recognized role in the diagnosis of cardiomyopathies. ICE has acquired an essential role in choosing the best sampling site, confirming the adequate position of the bioptome, and avoiding complications. The integration with EVM systems provides a complementary perspective, allowing visualization of diseased areas of myocardium displayed as regions of low or delayed/fragmented potentials. This combined approach, EVM and ICE, by integrating physiology and anatomy, enables the operator to visualize the best area(s) to sample, thus increasing the diagnostic yield of EMB, while at the same time reducing complications. This technique has proven to significantly increase the diagnostic yield of EMB in observational studies. Prospective trials are warranted to establish its superiority compared with the conventional fluoroscopy-guided approach, and to confirm its relevance in enabling a patient-tailored approach to cardiomyopathies in the era of personalized cardiovascular medicine.

CLINICS CARE POINTS

- EMB represents an important tool in the management of patients with ventricular arrhythmias and nonischemic cardiomyopathy.

- The combined use of ICE and EVM has allowed significant increase in the diagnostic yield of EMB.

- EVM enables (1) identification of the regional distribution of disease processes, displayed as low-voltage regions in a color-coded map; and (2) visualization of the bioptome in rapport with the surrounding structures.

- ICE enables the operator to choose the best sampling site, confirm the adequate position of the bioptome, and avoid complications.

DISCLOSURES

Dr. Dello Russo has received consulting fees and honoraria from Biosense Webster. Dr. Tondo has received consulting fees and honoraria from

Abbott Medical Inc., Medtronic, Boston Scientific, and Biosense Webster, and serves as a member of EU Medtronic Advisory Board and Boston Scientific Advisory Board.

SUPPLEMENTARY DATA

Supplementary data related to this article can be found online at https://doi.org/10.1016/j.ccep.2021.02.005.

REFERENCES

1. Avella A, d'Amati G, Pappalardo A, et al. Diagnostic value of endomyocardial biopsy guided by electroanatomic voltage mapping in arrhythmogenic right ventricular cardiomyopathy/dysplasia. J Cardiovasc Electrophysiol 2008;19(11):1127–34.

2. Pieroni M, Dello Russo A, Marzo F, et al. High prevalence of myocarditis mimicking arrhythmogenic right ventricular cardiomyopathy differential diagnosis by electroanatomic mapping-guided endomyocardial biopsy. J Am Coll Cardiol 2009;53(8):681–9.

3. Casella M, Pizzamiglio F, Dello Russo A, et al. Feasibility of combined unipolar and bipolar voltage maps to improve sensitivity of endomyocardial biopsy. Circ Arrhythm Electrophysiol 2015;8(3):625–32.

4. Casella M, Dello Russo A, Vettor G, et al. Electroanatomical mapping systems and intracardiac echo integration for guided endomyocardial biopsy. Expert Rev Med Devices 2017;14(8):609–19.

5. Casella M, Dello Russo A, Bergonti M, et al. Diagnostic yield of electroanatomic voltage mapping in guiding endomyocardial biopsies. Circulation 2020. https://doi.org/10.1161/CIRCULATIONAHA.120.046900.

6. Cooper LT, Baughman KL, Feldman AM, et al. The role of endomyocardial biopsy in the management of cardiovascular disease: a scientific statement from the American Heart Association, the American College of Cardiology, and the European Society of Cardiology. Endorsed by the Heart Failure Society of America and the Heart Failure Association of the European Society of Cardiology. Circulation 2007;28(24):3076–93.

7. Holzmann M, Nicko A, Kuhl U, et al. Complication rate of right ventricular endomyocardial biopsy via the femoral approach: a retrospective and prospective study analyzing 3048 diagnostic procedures over an 11-year period. Circulation 2008;118(17):1722–8.

8. Leone O, Veinot JP, Angelini A, et al. 2011 consensus statement on endomyocardial biopsy from the Association for European

Cardiovascular Pathology and the Society for Cardiovascular Pathology. Cardiovasc Pathol 2012;21(4):245–74.

9. Thiene G, Bruneval P, Veinot J, et al. Diagnostic use of the endomyocardial biopsy: a consensus statement. Virchows Arch 2013;463(1):1–5.

10. Towbin JA, McKenna WJ, Abrams DJ, et al. 2019 HRS expert consensus statement on evaluation, risk stratification, and management of arrhythmogenic cardiomyopathy. Hear Rhythm 2019;16(11):e301–72.

11. Marcus FI, McKenna WJ, Sherrill D, et al. Diagnosis of arrhythmogenic right ventricular cardiomyopathy/dysplasia: proposed modification of the task force criteria. Circulation 2010;121(13):1533–41.

12. Caforio ALP, Pankuweit S, Arbustini E, et al. Current state of knowledge on aetiology, diagnosis, management, and therapy of myocarditis: a position statement of the European Society of Cardiology Working Group on Myocardial and Pericardial Diseases. Eur Heart J 2013;34(33):2636–48, 2648a-2648d.

13. Birnie DH, Sauer WH, Bogun F, et al. HRS expert consensus statement on the diagnosis and management of arrhythmias associated with cardiac sarcoidosis. Hear Rhythm 2014;11(7):1305–23.

14. Enriquez A, Saenz LC, Rosso R, et al. Use of intracardiac echocardiography in interventional cardiology: working with the anatomy rather than fighting it. Circulation 2018;137(21):2278–94.

15. Zanobini M, Dello Russo A, Saccocci M, et al. Endomyocardial biopsy guided by intracardiac echocardiography as a key step in intracardiac mass diagnosis. BMC Cardiovasc Disord 2018;18(1):15.

16. Vaidya VR, Abudan AA, Vasudevan K, et al. The efficacy and safety of electroanatomic mapping-guided endomyocardial biopsy: a systematic review. J Interv Card Electrophysiol 2018;53(1):63–71.

17. Corrado D, Basso C, Leoni L, et al. Three-dimensional electroanatomical voltage mapping and histologic evaluation of myocardial substrate in right ventricular outflow tract tachycardia. J Am Coll Cardiol 2008;51(7):731–9.

18. Khaykin Y, Skanes A, Whaley B, et al. Real-time integration of 2D intracardiac echocardiography and 3D electroanatomical mapping to guide ventricular tachycardia ablation. Hear Rhythm 2008;5(10):1396–402.

19. Corrado D, Basso C, Leoni L, et al. Three-dimensional electroanatomic voltage mapping increases accuracy of diagnosing arrhythmogenic right ventricular cardiomyopathy/dysplasia. Circulation 2005;111(23):3042–50.

20. Polin GM, Haqqani H, Tzou W, et al. Endocardial unipolar voltage mapping to identify epicardial substrate in arrhythmogenic right ventricular cardiomyopathy/dysplasia. Hear Rhythm 2011;8(1): 76–83.

21. Schleifer JW, Manocha KK, Asirvatham SJ, et al. Feasibility of performing radiofrequency catheter ablation and endomyocardial biopsy in the same setting. Am J Cardiol 2018;121(11):1373–9.

22. Killu AM, Mehta N, Zheng Q, et al. Endomyocardial biopsy at the time of ablation or device implantation. J Interv Card Electrophysiol 2018; 52(2):163–9.

Epicardial and Coronary Sinus Echocardiography

Nicholas Palmeri, MD[a], Andre D'Avila, MD, PhD[a], Eduardo B. Saad, MD, PhD[b],*

KEYWORDS

- Pericardial access • Catheter-based ultrasonography • Intracardiac echocardiography
- Epicardial ablation • Electrophysiology • Echocardiography

KEY POINTS

- Intrapericardial echocardiography and coronary sinus echocardiography are used to obtain unique views of specific heart structures without the typical anatomic constraints of other forms of echocardiography.
- Obtaining views from within the pericardium is safe when performed by operators familiar with pericardial access.
- Views obtained from the pericardial space are used to visualize important near-frame and far-frame cardiac structures without catheter interference or shadowing.
- Familiarity with advanced imaging techniques is important for interventionalists performing complex ablation procedures.

 Video content accompanies this article at http://www.cardiacep.theclinics.com.

INTRODUCTION

Advances in echocardiographic technology have been essential to the facilitation of novel therapeutics in cardiac electrophysiology (EP). In addition to transthoracic echocardiography and transesophageal echocardiography (TEE), catheter-based ultrasonography is an important tool that has become common in the EP laboratory.[1] Intracardiac echocardiography (ICE) is routinely used and plays an important role in EP procedures, particularly for transseptal puncture and left atrial access.[2]

Other advantages of ICE, even compared with TEE, are increasingly appreciated, including its utility in identifying critical structures with high resolution, in real-time, without radiation.[3,4] ICE is increasingly used to evaluate the left atrium and left atrial appendage for thrombus[5–7] given its close proximity to structures in which ICE can be safely manipulated,[8] and ICE seems to have similar accuracy in identifying thrombus compared with TEE, based on basic science studies.[9] ICE may be even better than TEE at distinguishing clot characteristics and perhaps composition.[10] Definition of the esophageal borders is also critical to safe ablation within the left atrium, and ICE is capable of reliably visualizing the esophagus.[11,12] In the future, ICE may supplant TEE entirely.[13,14] The cardiac electrophysiologist can elegantly control the acquisition of images during EP procedures, and the utility of ICE imaging to monitor and evaluate for complications during EP procedures is one of its great strengths.[2,15] In fact, a recent contemporary study involving more than 100,000 ablation procedures showed that ICE nonuse was the single most important predictor of cardiac perforation during atrial fibrillation ablation, portending a nearly five-fold increase in risk.[16]

[a] Beth Israel Deaconess Medical Center, 185 Pilgrim Road, Boston, MA 02215, USA; [b] Cardiac Arrhythmia and Pacing, Center for Atrial Fibrillation - Hospital Pró-Cardíaco and Hospital Samaritano Botafogo, Rio de Janeiro, RJ, Brazil
* Corresponding author. Rua Visconde de Piraja 351/623, Ipanema, Rio de Janeiro, RJ 22470-001, Brazil.
E-mail address: eduardobsaad@hotmail.com

Card Electrophysiol Clin 13 (2021) 393–398
https://doi.org/10.1016/j.ccep.2021.03.003

Although ICE is the most common application of catheter-based ultrasound, the same instruments can also be introduced outside of the intravascular space. Intrapericardial echocardiography (IPE), also known as percutaneous intrapericardial cardiac echocardiography, is a means of using catheter-based ultrasonography to examine cardiac structures during EP interventions by introducing the same catheters used for ICE into the pericardial space. Coronary sinus echocardiography (CSE) is a variant of ICE that uses the epicardial vantage point afforded by the coronary venous system to obtain images in a similar fashion. Although experience is essential to the safe acquisition of such images, these techniques have a role in select settings.[1]

Using IPE allows visualizations of the heart in virtually any orientation, unencumbered by the anatomic limitations of transthoracic echocardiography, TEE, or even ICE. Moreover, the pericardial space offers an access point for imaging without concern for interference with other mapping or ablation catheters. CSE offers good catheter stability with excellent visualization of cardiac structures that are important to the practicing electrophysiologist. In this way, those trained in these techniques can manipulate catheters unbounded by conventional anatomic limitations to visualize virtually any cardiac structure, even in cases when other imaging modalities fail. As the epicardial approach to ablation expands, experience with IPE and CSE will likely become more important in the EP laboratory.

TECHNIQUE FOR PERICARDIAL ACCESS AND INTRODUCTION OF ULTRASOUND CATHETERS

Before obtaining images, access to the pericardial space must be obtained, usually in the absence of pericardial effusion. This has been described previously,[17] but briefly, it is accomplished through a subxiphoid approach using a Tuohy needle directed toward the left scapula and advanced into the space of Larrey. Contrast injection confirms entry into the pericardial space, and a soft guidewire is inserted. An introducer sheath can then be inserted over the wire into the pericardial space. The introducer sheath is directed based on the initial access approach, either toward the inferior aspect of the heart (steep approach, >45° angle) or toward the anterior aspect of the heart (shallow approach, <45° angle).

Once access has been established, the ultrasound catheter is advanced into the pericardial space through the introducer sheath using fluoroscopic guidance (Video 1). The pericardial

anatomy is complex, and although there are essentially no areas of pericardial reflection in the anterior portion of the pericardium, folding serous layers of pericardium create boundaries in the form of recesses on the posterior surface. Because many important structures of the heart are posterior, manipulating ultrasound catheters in this area is often necessary, and these recesses provide support for positioning. Thus, there are several stable approaches from which to visualize the heart in a variety of orientations.

Placing the catheter in the lateral-posterior aspect of the pericardial space with the ultrasound beam directed anteriorly and to the right provides a longitudinal four-chamber view of the heart (**Fig. 1**, Video 2). The left ventricle (LV) is near to the catheter with the right ventricle (RV) positioned deep to the catheter. This affords views of the LV cavity and papillary muscles, which is advantageous when performing ablation in the LV. Rotation and deflection of the catheter in this position within the pericardium can generate short-axis views of the LV, and images in this orientation are helpful to safely and effectively deliver ablation energy to the papillary muscles. The coronary vasculature can also be visualized from this vantage to safely perform epicardial ablation. Direction of the catheter superiorly into the region of the transverse sinus is useful for visualizing basal structures, such as the left atrium and mitral annulus.

With the catheter located in the anterior portion of the pericardium, the operator can manipulate the catheter more freely (Video 3). This is used for short-axis views of the LV and RV for target ablation. Advancing the catheter superiorly is useful for imaging of the RV outflow tract and ascending aorta with high image quality. Inferior views are used to visualize right atrial structures, including the right atrial appendage, and to visualize intravascular and intracardiac catheter position within the inferior vena cava and right atrium.

Although complications are theoretically possible while accessing the pericardial space, this is rare.[18] Typically, if bleeding into the pericardium occurs early after pericardial access, it is frequently not hemodynamically significant. If a small volume accumulates during the procedure or if an effusion persists, it is easily drained through the same access point at the end of the case. Active bleeding from an epicardial vessel can result in continued accumulation of blood products into the pericardium and may require surgical repair. Bleeding at the end of a procedure is worrisome, and it is also possible that a major complication, such as a "double RV puncture," may not be evident until the end of the procedure. Despite

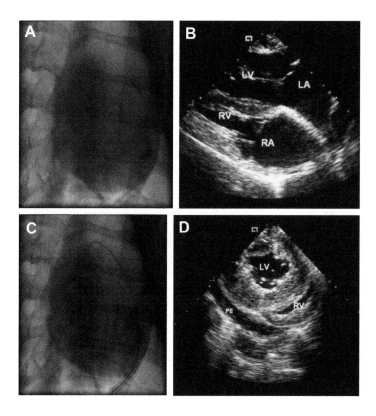

Fig. 1. IPE catheter positions. Positioning of the ultrasound catheter in the pericardial space with visualization of right atrial and right ventricular structures and the right ventricular outflow tract and the tricuspid valve from an anterior approach (A). Posterolateral view with the catheter positioned superiorly. (B) Posterolateral four-chamber view with the LV in the near field and RV and RA in the far field. (C) Anterior view of the LV. (D) Short-axis view of the LV with visualization of the mitral apparatus and papillary muscles. See accompanying online videos; some images adapted from Rodrigues and colleagues.[20] LA, left atrium; LV, left ventricle; PE, pericardial effusion; RA, right atrium; RV, right ventricle.

these potential complications, for those experienced with the techniques of epicardial access, IPE is a safe tool for imaging.

DESCRIPTIONS OF INTRAPERICARDIAL ECHOCARDIOGRAPHY AND CORONARY SINUS ECHOCARDIOGRAPHY VIEWS IN THE LITERATURE

Although descriptions of IPE/percutaneous intrapericardial cardiac echocardiography are rare, they have been available for more than a decade.[1] The technique was only made possible following two important advances: the development of modern catheter-based ultrasonography and pericardial access methods described previously. By itself, ICE has been a major innovation in EP,[19] but IPE and CSE are variations that bear special consideration.

A basic strategy of introducing ultrasound catheters into the pericardial space was first described in 2004 in an experimental setting in animals.[20] Ultrasound-based catheters used for ICE were inserted into the pericardial space under fluoroscopic guidance as described previously. The tip of the catheter was easily manipulated in the pericardial space, but simultaneously, stability was excellent because of the natural support provided by the pericardial sac. Control of the catheter was

also found to be superior to that afforded by ICE, because the operator was able to manipulate the catheter closer to the access point with a shorter length of catheter in the body.

The authors describe two major viewpoints from the posterior and anterior aspects of the pericardium. From the posterior perspective, the ultrasound catheter contacted the posterior wall of the LV. A longitudinal four-chamber view of the heart was obtained with the posterior wall of the LV and posteromedial papillary muscle in the foreground. Short-axis views were obtained with flexion and extension of the catheter at various levels to visualize the papillary muscles and the mitral valve annulus and surrounding structures. By directing the catheter more superiorly, the left atrium, right atrium, coronary sinus, and fossa ovalis could also be visualized.

In the anterior pericardium, the catheter was manipulated to contact the anterior wall of the LV and the RV free wall, and the right atrium. By rotating the catheter, the major blood vessels were visualized including the bodies and ostia of the inferior and superior vena cava, the aorta and LV outflow tract, and the pulmonary trunk and RV outflow tract. The coronary arteries were able to be visualized mid-field in the short-axis view, caused in part by the limited visualization of the near field with ultrasound-based catheters. This is important when choosing a location for ablation in the epicardial space. Each of these views has its clinical application for the electrophysiologist for assisting in complex EP interventions.

In humans, IPE has been described in 10 patients undergoing epicardial catheter ablation. Most were for Ventricular Tachycardia, although the technique was also used for accessory pathway ablation.[21] Other echocardiography techniques were also compared with IPE in this study, including ICE and TEE. It seemed that although images were overall similar, IPE had the advantage of less catheter interaction compared with ICE. The authors also attempted to correlate measured voltages with the function of the tissues as assessed by IPE; they found that lower voltages correlated with less robust contraction and higher voltages correlated with normal contraction.

Positioning of the catheter in this study was somewhat different from that described in animals previously. The authors described optimal stability while positioning the catheters in the oblique and transverse sinuses. Views obtained from the transverse sinus were used to visualize the aorta and pulmonary trunk. A posterior view from the oblique

sinus provided good visualization of the papillary muscles. The authors even describe changing their ablation strategy based on visualization of a calcified papillary muscle.

CSE has been described sporadically in the literature. Although more constrained by anatomy, stable positioning of the ultrasound catheter within the coronary sinus offers excellent views of the left atrium, left atrial appendage (**Fig. 2**), LV, and mitral annulus. Use of this position has been described for visualization of the left atrial appendage during implantation of left atrial appendage occlusion devices.[19,22]

This position offers excellent views during atrial fibrillation ablations, particularly for pulmonary vein isolation and ablation along the left atrial roof (see **Fig. 2**C, D). Ablation of the posterior mitral isthmus is one scenario in which CSE can be critical to resolve anatomic variants in important structures, such as the left circumflex artery.[23] Another variation on this perspective, almost the reverse of CSE, is manipulation of the ICE catheter within the body of the left atrium to visualize the CS.[24] This technique affords similar views of the coronary anatomy and of the mitral isthmus.

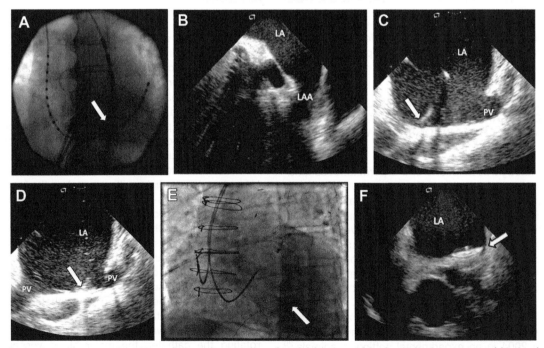

Fig. 2. CSE catheter positioning and views. Positioning of ICE catheters within the CS body permits stable visualization of various structures. (*A*) ICE catheter (*arrow*) positioned in the CS in a patient undergoing PVI. (*B*) Visualization of the LAA and exclusion of LAA thrombus. (*C*) Visualization of the circular mapping catheter (*arrow*) being manipulated in the LA roof, between the two superior PVs. (*D*) Direct visualization of an RFA catheter (*arrow*) delivering a linear radiofrequency lesion in the LA roof. (*E*) ICE catheter (*arrow*) positioned in the CS in a patient undergoing LAA occlusion (ACP device). (*F*) Visualization of the LAA with the occlusion device in place (*arrow*) with excellent resolution. See online supplement for full videos. Ao, aorta; CS, coronary sinus; LA, left atrium; LAA, left atrial appendage; PV, pulmonary vein; PVI, pulmonary vein isolation; RFA, radiofrequency ablation.

Clearly, ultrasound-based catheters provide a variety of perspectives to view critical structures.

Applications of IPE and CSE are likely to expand as technology evolves. A novel forward-facing catheter-based ultrasound probe that can simultaneously deliver radiofrequency ablation has been described and tested.[25] In an experimental porcine model, the catheter was introduced into the pericardium and manipulated to visualize various structures. These technologies could become more commonly used for epicardial procedures.

SUMMARY

Innovations in catheter-based technologies continue to expand the ability of the cardiac electrophysiologist to better visualize the structures of the heart. In turn, this provides greater opportunity to safely deliver therapies to treat and control arrhythmias according to their unique anatomic origins. Among these innovations, the use of IPE and CSE to image cardiac structures is an important technique, especially as epicardial procedures become more commonplace.

Although descriptions of this technique are limited, introduction of imaging catheters into the pericardium is a natural application of pericardial access. For those familiar with the technique, IPE is a safe imaging option that provides unprecedented angles from which to visualize cardiac structures. Adding this skill to one's arsenal further expands the reach and scope of imaging techniques for the cardiac electrophysiologist.

CLINICS CARE POINTS

- Intrapericardial echocardiography (IPE) and coronary sinus echocardiography (CSE) are techniques that take advantage of the unique vantages of the pericardium.
- IPE and CSE are useful for visualizing cardiac structures and avoiding complications during EP procedures.
- Posterior views are obtained with stable catheter position, but views of the heart are obtained from a variety of perspectives in the pericardium.
- IPE is a safe technique that may be an important tool for clinicians performing complex ablations, particularly in cases performed via the epicardial approach.

DISCLOSURE

None.

SUPPLEMENTARY DATA

Supplementary data related to this article can be found online at https://doi.org/10.1016/j.ccep.2021.03.003.

REFERENCES

1. Hijazi ZM, Shivkumar K, Sahn DJ. Intracardiac echocardiography during interventional and electrophysiological cardiac catheterization. Circulation 2009; 119(4):587–96.
2. Ren J-F, Marchlinski FE. Utility of intracardiac echocardiography in left heart ablation for tachyarrhythmias. Echocardiography 2007;24(5):533–40.
3. Anter E, Silverstein J, Tschabrunn CM, et al. Comparison of intracardiac echocardiography and transesophageal echocardiography for imaging of the right and left atrial appendages. Heart Rhythm 2014;11(11):1890–7.
4. Desimone CV, Asirvatham SJ. ICE imaging of the left atrial appendage. J Cardiovasc Electrophysiol 2014; 25(11):1272–4.
5. Sriram CS, Banchs JE, Moukabary T, et al. Detection of left atrial thrombus by intracardiac echocardiography in patients undergoing ablation of atrial fibrillation. J Interv Card Electrophysiol 2015;43(3): 227–36.
6. Baran J, Stec S, Pilichowska-Paszkiet E, et al. Intracardiac echocardiography for detection of thrombus in the left atrial appendage: comparison with transesophageal echocardiography in patients undergoing ablation for atrial fibrillation: the Action-Ice I Study. Circ Arrhythm Electrophysiol 2013;6(6): 1074–81.
7. Saksena S, Sra J, Jordaens L, et al. A prospective comparison of cardiac imaging using intracardiac echocardiography with transesophageal echocardiography in patients with atrial fibrillation: the intracardiac echocardiography guided cardioversion helps interventional procedures study. Circ Arrhythm Electrophysiol 2010;3(6):571–7.
8. Nishiyama T, Katsumata Y, Inagawa K, et al. Visualization of the left atrial appendage by phased-array intracardiac echocardiography from the pulmonary artery in patients with atrial fibrillation. Europace 2015;17(4):546–51.
9. Hutchinson MD, Jacobson JT, Michele JJ, et al. A comparison of intracardiac and transesophageal echocardiography to detect left atrial appendage thrombus in a swine model. J Interv Card Electrophysiol 2010;27(1):3–7.
10. Baran J, Zaborska B, Piotrowski R, et al. Intracardiac echocardiography for verification for left atrial

appendage thrombus presence detected by transe-sophageal echocardiography: the ActionICE II study. Clin Cardiol 2017;40(7):450–4.

11. Kenigsberg DN, Lee BP, Grizzard JD, et al. Accuracy of intracardiac echocardiography for assessing the esophageal course along the posterior left atrium: a comparison to magnetic resonance imaging. J Cardiovasc Electrophysiol 2007;18(2):169–73.

12. Bunch TJ, May HT, Crandall BG, et al. Intracardiac ultrasound for esophageal anatomic assessment and localization during left atrial ablation for atrial fibrillation. J Cardiovasc Electrophysiol 2013;24(1):33–9.

13. Themistoclakis S, Rossillo A, Bonso A, et al. Intracardiac echocardiography for implantation of LAA occlusion devices: a further step toward the ICE era? Heart Rhythm 2007;4(5):572–4.

14. Goya M, Frame D, Gache L, et al. The use of intracardiac echocardiography catheters in endocardial ablation of cardiac arrhythmia: meta-analysis of efficiency, effectiveness, and safety outcomes. J Cardiovasc Electrophysiol 2020;31(3):664–73.

15. Jongbloed MRM. Clinical applications of intracardiac echocardiography in interventional procedures. Heart 2005;91(7):981–90.

16. Friedman DJ, Pokorney SD, Ghanem A, et al. Predictors of cardiac perforation with catheter ablation of atrial fibrillation. JACC Clin Electrophysiol 2020;6(6):636–45.

17. Aryana A, Tung R, d'Avila A. Percutaneous epicardial approach to catheter ablation of cardiac arrhythmias. JACC Clin Electrophysiol 2020;6(1):1–20.

18. Aryana A, d'Avila A. Epicardial approach for cardiac electrophysiology procedures. J Cardiovasc Electrophysiol 2020;31(1):345–59.

19. Enriquez A, Saenz LC, Rosso R, et al. Use of intracardiac echocardiography in interventional cardiology: working with the anatomy rather than fighting it. Circulation 2018;137(21):2278–94.

20. Rodrigues ACT, d'Avila A, Houghtaling C, et al. Intrapericardial echocardiography: a novel catheter-based approach to cardiac imaging. J Am Soc Echocardiogr 2004;17(3):269–74.

21. Horowitz BN, Vaseghi M, Mahajan A, et al. Percutaneous intrapericardial echocardiography during catheter ablation: a feasibility study. Heart Rhythm 2006;3(11):1275–82.

22. Ho ICK, Neuzil P, Mraz T, et al. Use of intracardiac echocardiography to guide implantation of a left atrial appendage occlusion device (PLAATO). Heart Rhythm 2007;4(5):567–71.

23. West JJ, Norton PT, Kramer CM, et al. Characterization of the mitral isthmus for atrial fibrillation ablation using intracardiac ultrasound from within the coronary sinus. Heart Rhythm 2008;5(1):19–27.

24. Flautt TJ, Spangler AL, Prather JW, et al. A novel mapping and ablation strategy of the mitral isthmus using intracardiac echocardiography in the left atrium. Hear Case Rep 2018;5(2):80–2.

25. Stephens DN, Truong UT, Nikoozadeh A, et al. First in vivo use of a capacitive micromachined ultrasound transducer array-based imaging and ablation catheter. J Ultrasound Med 2012;31(2):247–56.

Intracardiac Echocardiography to Guide Non-fluoroscopic Electrophysiology Procedures

Josef Kautzner, MD, PhD[a,b,*], Jana Haskova, MD[a], Frantisek Lehar, MD, PhD[a,c]

KEYWORDS

- Electroanatomic mapping • Electrophysiology procedures • Intracardiac echocardiography
- Fluoroscopy

KEY POINTS

- Advantages of intracardiac echocardiography (ICE) in electrophysiology procedures include the ease of use, no need for general anesthesia or deep sedation and the possibility of the adjustment of the imaging view according to locate mapping and ablation catheters.
- ICE may be used with or without electroanatomical mapping system for non-fluoroscopical conventional ablation procedures, especially for guidance of catheter ablation of cavotricuspid isthmus in atrial flutter.
- ICE allows safe and reproducible transseptal puncture.
- ICE is an important tool for guidance in complex ablation procedures, often together with electroanatomical mapping system.
- Assessment of the extent and location myocardial substrate for ventricular arrhythmias is another domain of ICE.

 Video content accompanies this article at http://www.cardiacep.theclinics.com.

The traditional way of performing interventional electrophysiology procedures (EP) relied solely on fluoroscopic guidance. However, the situation has changed over time, mainly for 3 reasons. First, extensive radiation exposure in the early period of catheter ablations has resulted in efforts for a significant reduction of radiation burden, both for the patient and the staff.[1] Second, the need for visualization of relevant anatomic structures in complex catheter ablation procedures (eg, anatomy of the pulmonary veins in ablation of atrial fibrillation or papillary muscles in ablation of ectopic foci from this region) led to the introduction of electroanatomic mapping (EAM) systems and intracardiac echocardiography (ICE). Third, the risk of musculoskeletal complications among operators due to prolonged use of lead aprons has encouraged the search for non-fluoroscopic approach.

Over time, the use of EAM systems and optional co-registration of electroanatomical maps with 3-dimensional computed tomography (CT) or MR images has become widespread for all complex procedures. However, the main progress has occurred due to the implementation of ICE. Online

---

This work was supported by the Research Grant of the Ministry of Health, Czech Republic— Conceptual development of research organization ("Institute for Clinical and Experimental Medicine—IKEM, IN 00023001").

[a] Department of Cardiology, Institute for Clinical and Experimental Medicine, Prague, Czech Republic;
[b] Palacky University Medical School, Olomouc, Czech Republic; [c] Department of Internal Medicine 1–Cardioangiology, St Anne's University Hospital, Brno, Czech Republic
* Corresponding author. Department of Cardiology, Institute for Clinical and Experimental Medicine, Vídeňská 1958/9, Prague 4 14021, Czech Republic.
E-mail address: joka@ikem.cz

imaging allows guiding complex procedures together with EAM systems either with minimal fluoroscopic exposure or with zero fluoroscopy. Still, many operators rely heavily on fluoroscopic guidance during EP interventions. The following text describes the clinical utility of ICE in non-fluoroscopic EP procedures.

TYPES OF NON-FLUOROSCOPIC PROCEDURES

Non-fluoroscopic procedures can be divided into conventional or complex ablations. Conventional ablations comprise most frequently catheter ablation for atrioventricular nodal reentry (AVNRT), catheter ablation of accessory pathways, focal atrial tachycardias, and typical atrial flutter. In this category, most procedures can be done safely without ICE guidance, just with the support of the EAM system. Especially the cases without the need for transseptal (TS) puncture. Some centers use the EAM-based, non-fluoroscopic approach also for ablation of idiopathic ventricular premature beats (VPBs) or ventricular tachycardias (VT).[2–10]

Procedures requiring TS puncture may be performed safely without fluoroscopic guidance only under ICE guidance.

Complex ablations require either the TS approach or an EAM system to support the mapping and ablation. A typical example of complex ablation that can be performed without fluoroscopy guidance is atrial fibrillation (AF). In this case, ICE appears to be a mandatory imaging tool. Ventricular arrhythmias in structural heart disease are ablated with zero fluoroscopic approaches less frequently. This can be attributed to various reasons, including limitations of supportive imaging tools, the complexity of ventricular anatomy, limited experience of the operators, and the presence of intracardiac devices with the risk of lead dislocation. However, several groups published data on the use of ICE and EAM systems also in subjects with these specific VTs.

THE ADVANTAGES OF INTRACARDIAC ECHOCARDIOGRAPHY

ICE is the most practical method for online imaging during many interventional procedures.[11] The main advantages include ease of use, no need for general anesthesia or deep sedation, and the possibility of adjustment of the imaging view. The quality of imaging is variable in different patients, but the proximity to cardiac structure allows good visualization of the relevant structures, often far better than in transesophageal echocardiography. It also can display the regions that are shielded by the artificial prostheses and/or occluders. Compared with rotational ultrasound catheter, which has limited maneuverability and depth of imaging, phased-array systems are very versatile and provide the whole spectrum of 2-dimensional images, including color-coded or pulsed wave Doppler. In addition, they allow adjustment of ultrasound frequency to optimize imaging quality. The ICE catheter is typically advanced from the femoral vein into the right atrium, right ventricle, or other chambers, depending on the need for visualization. The advancement of the ICE probe can be monitored without the need for fluoroscopy and imaging within iliac veins and/or inferior vena cava enable the introduction of diagnostic and ablation catheters. ICE imaging at the level of the right atrium enables the safe introduction of wires into the superior vena cava and subsequent zero fluoroscopy TS puncture.

CATHETER ABLATION OF CONVENTIONAL ARRHYTHMIAS

As mentioned previously, most non-fluoroscopic conventional ablations can be performed without ICE guidance. Nevertheless, some centers explored the possibility of using ICE instead of the EAM system or in parallel to it.

Intracardiac Echocardiography–Guided Catheter Ablation of Atrioventricular Nodal Reentry

The feasibility and safety of the cryothermal catheter ablation of this arrhythmia guided solely by ICE were investigated by Luani and colleagues.[12] A total of 25 subjects were studied and all catheters were placed by ICE guidance. Finally, 80% had typical AVNRT, which was ablated without the need for fluoroscopy. Among the advantages of ICE over the 3-dimensional (3D) EAM system, the investigators mentioned direct visualization of the structures and catheter tip and its contact with the tissue.

Intracardiac Echocardiography–Guided Catheter Ablation of Atrial Flutter

Although ICE was used in a small series of patients already in 2003, routine guidance of ablation is not generally used.[13] Reports on the use of ICE for flutter ablation without fluoroscopy are part of studies on the use of ICE guidance in the whole spectrum of arrhythmias.[14] We believe that the knowledge of the particular anatomy of the cavotricuspid isthmus is more important than the use of the EAM system. Our earlier analysis showed that certain anatomic variants cause difficulties in achievement block on the isthmus (Unpublished data, 2006). One of the

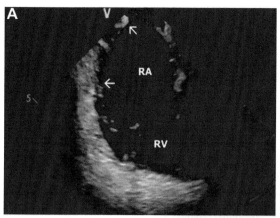
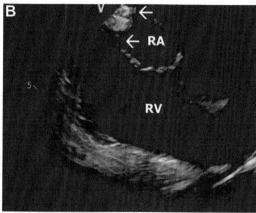
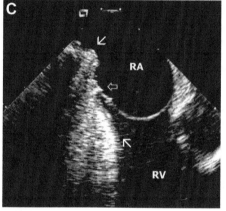

Fig. 1. ICE depiction of the hypermobile cavotricuspid isthmus (*A*) in ventricular diastole and (*B*) in ventricular systole (closure of the tricuspid valve). *Arrows* show the length of the isthmus in different phases of the cardiac cycle. (*C*) Illustration of a maneuver with the ablation catheter to stabilize the tissue in case of the hypermobile isthmus (*arrows* mark the length of the isthmus, *empty arrow* shows the tip of the catheter). RA, right atrium; RV, right ventricle.

most intriguing is the so-called hypermobile isthmus. In such a case, the tissue of the isthmus is loose and moving with every heartbeat, compressing and extending from end-diastole to systole. This anatomic variant was observed in our pilot study on 96 patients (54 men, mean age 54.5 ± 11.5 years) in 9% of cases (**Fig. 1**, Video 1). Another specific isthmus morphology that can make the procedure difficult is the prominent Eustachian ridge (more than 8 mm). This type was recognized in 24% of subjects (**Fig. 2**). In some rare cases, the anatomy of the isthmus is completely abnormal (**Fig. 3**, Video 2).

Intracardiac Echocardiography–Guided Catheter Ablation of Accessory Pathways

A report on successful ablation of a case series of right-sided accessory pathways using ICE and the EAM system was published recently.[15] ICE imaging allowed reproducible placement of the ablation catheter below the cusps of the tricuspid valve to achieve better stability. We have similar experience with this strategy (**Fig. 4**, Video 3).

Intracardiac Echocardiography–Guided Catheter Ablation of Idiopathic Ventricular Tachycardia or Ventricular Premature Beats

A recent study on the use of the EAM system and ICE to ablate idiopathic VT reported the results in 19

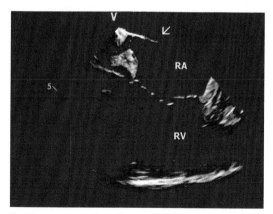

Fig. 2. An example of a very prominent Eustachian ridge (*arrow*). RA, right atrium; RV, right ventricle.

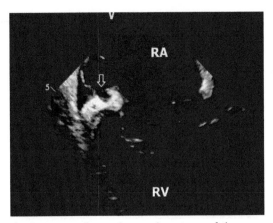

Fig. 3. A case of very abnormal anatomy of the cavo-tricuspid isthmus which is very short and perpendicular to the valve with a small recess (*empty arrow*). The rest of the tissue toward the inferior vena cava is just a floppy membrane without any musculature and electrograms. RA, right atrium; RV, right ventricle.

patients. No fluoroscopy was used in any procedural phase. The acute success rate was 100% without complications. After a mean follow-up of 18 ± 4 months, recurrences occurred in 2 patients.[16]

PROCEDURES REQUIRING TRANSSEPTAL PUNCTURE
Zero Fluoroscopy Transseptal Puncture

TS puncture could be performed without fluoroscopy using a variety of techniques and tools by individual operators. Generally, 2 different technical approaches for TS are used.[17]

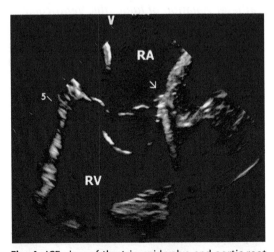

Fig. 4. ICE view of the tricuspid valve and aortic root showing catheter tip embedded underneath the anterior leaflet of the tricuspid valve (*arrow*) in a young female with an anterior accessory pathway. RA, right atrium; RV, right ventricle.

One strategy is similar to conventional, fluoroscopy-guided TS puncture. Instead of fluoroscopy, ICE is used to navigate the sheath with the TS needle into the fossa ovalis. The procedure starts with placement of the guide-wires in the superior vena cava and delivery of the long sheath into it (either nonsteerable, like SL1, or steerable, like Agilis, St Jude Medical-Abbott) under ICE control (**Fig. 5**, Video 4). After the introduction of the TS needle, the sheath-needle assembly is pulled down similar to the fluoroscopy-guided procedure until the tip of the sheath is recognized on the ICE image in the fossa ovalis. After optimization of the puncture site (more posterior for ablation of pulmonary veins, more anterior for accessory pathway mapping or mapping of the left ventricle) with appropriate tenting (**Fig. 6**A), the TS needle is advanced briskly from the dilator, and penetration across the septum is visualized by a small puff of the physiologic solution (see **Fig. 6**B). The dilator, together with the TS sheath itself, is carefully advanced over the needle into the left atrium under continuous ICE guidance. For some procedures, one puncture is enough. Other procedures require the introduction of another sheath. Some operators use only one puncture and pull back the sheath into the right atrium, retaining the wire through the puncture hole and anchoring in the pulmonary vein (**Fig. 7**A). Subsequently, they introduce through the second sheath the ablation catheter into the hole in the fossa ovalis and push the sheath into the left atrium. The other sheath with the dilator is then introduced over the wire into the left atrium. In one of our teams, we have used for many years a double TS puncture for AF procedures.[18] After the first puncture, we introduce the circular catheter into one of the pulmonary veins (see **Fig. 7**B). This stabilizes the fossa ovalis and the second TS puncture is usually easier.

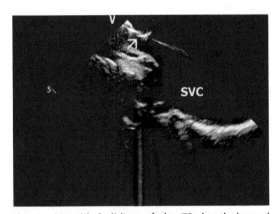

Fig. 5. ICE-guided sliding of the TS sheath (*arrow*) over the guidewire into the superior vena cava (SVC).

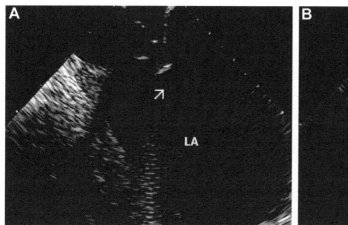
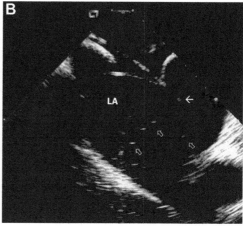

Fig. 6. (A) Tenting of the TS needle in the middle part of the fossa ovalis before puncture (*arrow*). (B) Needle tip crossed fossa ovalis (*arrow*) and this is confirmed by microbubbles from injected saline (*empty arrows*). LA, left atrium.

The second strategy differs in a way that after the introduction of the TS sheath into the right atrium, the ablation catheter is advanced through it and the volumetric map of the right atrium and coronary sinus ostium is performed.[19] The ablation catheter is then positioned onto the fossa ovalis under ICE guidance, followed by advancement of the sheath over the ablation catheter until mild tenting is seen. The ablation catheter is then withdrawn with a continuing push of sheath to maintain tenting (**Fig. 8**). Subsequently, the dilator with the TS needle is introduced into the sheath. Once the tip of the dilator is visualized by ICE, the tenting of the septum is checked and the needle is advanced, and then the whole assembly into the left atrium.

CATHETER ABLATION OF COMPLEX ARRHYTHMIAS
Catheter Ablation of Atrial Fibrillation and Left Atrial Tachycardias

The ablation of AF is a complex procedure with many steps, irrespective of the technology used for ablation itself. The most important difference from conventional ablation is a need for 1 or 2 TS punctures. Besides, the identification of pulmonary venous ostia requires some form of imaging (**Fig. 9**, Video 5). Depending on the technology used, catheter manipulation in the left atrium also should be visualized. Zero fluoroscopy procedure guided only by ICE could be performed for cryoablation, that is, without the need for EAM.[20]

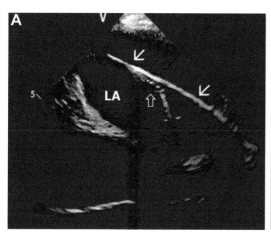
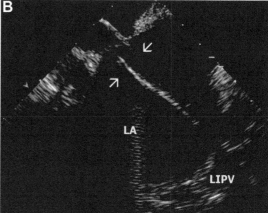

Fig. 7. (A) An example of a retained guidewire across the fossa ovalis (*arrows*) and introduction of the ablation catheter through the same puncture hole into the LA (*empty arrow*). (B) Double TS puncture with 2 sheaths introduced separately into the LA after anchoring the first one in the left inferior pulmonary vein with the circular mapping catheter. LA, left atrium; LIPV, left inferior pulmonary vein.

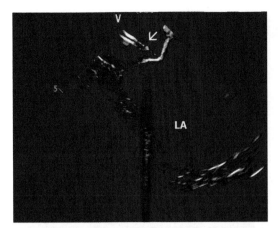

Fig. 8. The tip of the steerable sheath navigated to the center of fossa ovalis (arrow) by ablation catheter with the help of an electroanatomic mapping system and ICE. TS puncture is performed after the introduction of the needle with a dilator. LA, left atrium.

Similarly, the laser-balloon catheter could be manipulated only with the guidance of ICE. However, few available studies also used EAM together with ICE.[21–23] For conventional point-by-point ablation strategies, EAM is an important adjunct for understanding 3D anatomy and also for the assessment of voltages. It is also used for visualization of the guide-wires passing into the superior vena cava. At the same time, it enables monitoring of the introduction of the mapping catheter from the left femoral vein into the inferior vena cava and to the coronary sinus.

Left atrial geometry can be mapped using different approaches. One is to use a circular

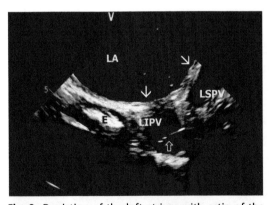

Fig. 9. Depiction of the left atrium with ostia of the left-sided pulmonary veins and the carina (arrows) between them and anteriorly located left appendage. A circular mapping catheter is introduced in the LIPV (empty arrow) and ablation catheter is located on the carina (between the arrows). LA, left atrium; E, esophagus; LIPV, LSPV, left inferior and left superior pulmonary vein, respectively.

catheter and Ensite NAVx to create the map of the pulmonary veins and the left atrial body under visual guidance by ICE.[24,25] A similar approach can be used with a sensor-enabled circular catheter with the CARTO EAM system.[26] Some operators prefer a point-by-point acquisition method with the ablation catheter with contact force-sensing capability (a 3.5-mm irrigated-tip Thermo-Cool Smart Touch [Biosense Webster Inc, Irvine, CA], or Tacticath [St Jude Medical – Abbott, St Paul, MN]).[27] Another option is to merge such an electroanatomical map with the prerequired CT or MR scan (or rotational angiography reconstruction) scan and used this 3D image for ablation.[28,29]

Others may prefer to use the ICE catheter with a magnetic sensor (CARTSOUND) and draw the contours of the left atrium and the pulmonary vein ostia, and build the 3D map in this way. The map can be merged with the CT or MR scan (or 3D reconstruction from rotational angiography) and used for subsequent ablation without the need for mapping of the atrium with the mapping catheter[30,31] (Fig. 10).

Another great advantage of ICE is the possibility of continuous monitoring for potential complications such as hemopericardium. One can detect this complication far before cardiac tamponade becomes manifest and perform pericardial drainage upfront (Figs. 11A,B).

Catheter Ablation of Ventricular Tachycardia

Sadek and colleagues[32] reported on non-fluoroscopic ablation supported by ICE in 80 patients, including 10 subjects with VT/VPB. Four patients had idiopathic arrhythmia and 6 VT in structural heart disease. They observed a modest learning curve and procedure duration in the last 10 cases was comparable to fluoroscopy-guided ablation. All patients with outflow-tract VPCs demonstrated no recurrence during follow-up, and the treatment success rate was 83% in patients with scar-mediated VTs. As most of these patients have intracardiac devices, the study focused also on visualization the leads before and after the procedure. Razminia and colleagues[26] published on a 5-year experience with non-fluoroscopic ablation supported by EAM and ICE. A total of 639 ablations in 500 patients were performed and 21.4% were for ventricular arrhythmias. Major complications occurred in 5 patients (1.0%); minor complications occurred in 3 patients (0.6%). Sánchez and colleagues[33] reported their single-center experience with a fluoroless approach using 3D EAM in all patients and ICE in 70.4% of patients. The study included a total of 10 ablation procedures for ventricular arrhythmias

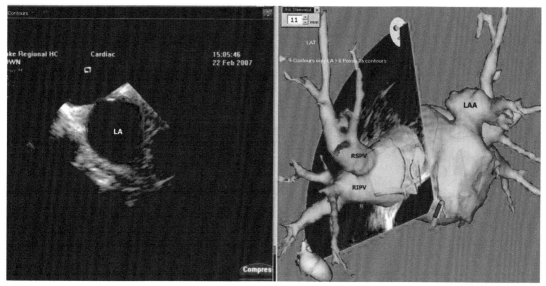

Fig. 10. An example of image integration for ablation in the LA using ICE imaging with CARTOSOUND. (*A*) Contours of the LA in one slice. (*B*) Merge of obtained contours in one ultrasound slice with CT angiogram of the left atrium and pulmonary veins (right anterior oblique view). LA, left atrium; LAA, left atrial appendage; RIPV, RSPV, right inferior and right superior pulmonary vein, respectively.

including VPCs and VTs with a mean procedure time of 150 minutes ± 45 minutes and no complications. A Slovenian group published recent data on 586 fluoroless ablation procedures, and 33 (5.6%) of them were for left-sided VT.[18] The overall procedural complication rate was 1.9% (11 of 586 procedures).

One of the additional advantages of ICE in ablation of VT in structural heart disease is the possibility to visualize the substrate and its extent in most cases (**Fig. 12**).

CATHETER ABLATION IN SPECIAL POPULATIONS

Fluoroless catheter ablation procedures may be of the utmost importance when it comes to specific patient subgroups such as pregnant women or children. In pregnant women, the avoidance of radiation exposure is especially critical during the first trimester of pregnancy because of the higher risk for fetal adverse effects. Data on the fluoroless approach are available from just a few case reports and case series (**Fig. 13**). The largest series was described by a group from Beijing.[34] Among 156 pregnant women with tachyarrhythmias, 28 received nonfluoroscopic catheter ablation with the support of the EAM system (CARTO). TS punctures were performed in 11 patients and were guided by ICE. There were 13 cases of ventricular arrhythmia. Other arrhythmias included AVNRT (n = 4), incessant atrial tachycardia (n = 6), and paroxysmal AF (n = 2), and arrhythmias due to

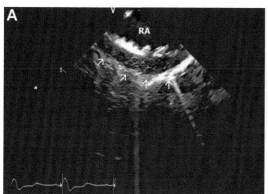
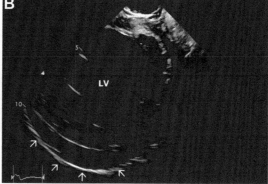

Fig. 11. (*A*) Separation around the right atrial wall (*arrows* mark the parietal pericardium). RA, right atrium. (*B*) Pathologic separation below the left ventricular wall (*arrows* mark the parietal pericardium). LV, left ventricle.

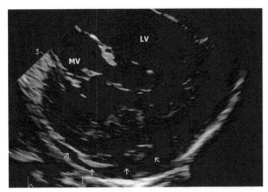

Fig. 12. ICE image of the LV from the right ventricle, showing the epicardial location of scar tissue in a patient with nonischemic cardiomyopathy and recurrent VTs. LV, left ventricle; MV, mitral valve.

accessory pathways (n = 3). During the later follow-up, all patients were free of arrhythmia, and all the infants were well developed.

Children and newborns are a special subpopulation with a higher lifelong cumulative risk of radiation-related morbidity. In these very young patients, minimal or zero fluoroscopy approaches, usually with the use of 3D EAM and ICE, have been implemented earlier and more rapidly than in adult patients.[35,36] This was possible because most of the cardiac arrhythmias observed in children are supraventricular tachycardia with a right-sided origin (>90% of cases are AVNRT), which can be easily treated with fluoroless procedures.

Recently, Žižek and colleagues[18] reported the results of successful non-fluoroscopic ablation guided by ICE and EAM system in 46 pediatric patients. This subgroup comprised 7.8% of all non-fluoroscopy procedures of the published cohort. Of those, 41 procedures were performed for accessory pathways, 4 for focal atrial tachycardias, and 1 for fascicular VT. Seven ablations (7 of 46, 15%) were performed in patients weighing less than 30 kg. The youngest patient was 4 years old and weighed 17 kg.

OUR EXPERIENCE WITH NON-FLUOROSCOPIC PROCEDURES

We initiated a zero fluoroscopy program in 2018. Our pilot study of 70 patients undergoing ablation for AF with ("X-ray group" - 35) and without ("ZeroFluoro" group - 35) fluoroscopy has documented the feasibility and safety of the non-fluoroscopic approach with a short learning curve. We observed no statistically significant difference in the total procedural time was (X-ray 132 minutes vs ZeroFluoro 143 minutes, $P = .20$). There was no need for fluoroscopy in the ZeroFluoro group, whereas in the X-ray group the average fluoroscopy time was 6.7 minutes (SD ± 4.3 minutes). The total radiofrequency delivery time was comparable in both groups (X-ray 2377 seconds vs ZeroFluoro 2346 seconds, $P = .91$). In all patients, isolation of the pulmonary veins was achieved. Only 2 complications were noted, both in the X-ray group (1 tamponade requiring pericardial drainage, 1 reactive pericardial effusion).

Since 2019, the non-fluoroscopic approach has become a routine for dedicated operators in our arrhythmia teams. Altogether, we performed

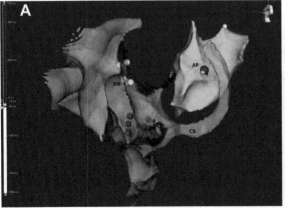
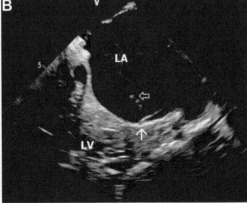

Fig. 13. (A) Minimalistic electroanatomical map of the right atrium with ostium of the coronary sinus and its course. Red tag annotates the site of ablation of the left lateral accessory pathway, the white area on the activation map depicts the earliest atrial activation during atypical AVNRT with ablations points around (left oblique view). HB, his bundle; SP, area od slow pathway; CS, coronary sinus; AP, site of ablation of the accessory pathway. (B) ICE view of the LA and mitral annulus with the tip of ablation catheter located laterally (arrow). Empty arrow depicts microbubbles from catheter irrigation. LA, left atrium; LV, left ventricle.

more than 368 zero fluoroscopy procedures: AF (n = 234), atypical flutter (n = 14), focal atrial tachycardia (n = 12), AVNRT (n = 82), typical flutter (n = 24), and accessory pathways (n = 2). Only 1 hemodynamically nonsignificant pericardial effusion has been observed over this period during ablation for AF.

LIMITATIONS OF NON-FLUOROSCOPIC APPROACH

Performing non-fluoroscopic catheter ablation of complex arrhythmias requires substantial experience and competency with ICE imaging. Therefore, operators interested in the non-fluoroscopic approach require training in ICE imaging and they should perform a series of cases with fluoroscopy back-up during each step of the procedure before transitioning completely. It is important to be competent with fluoroscopic imaging to allow "rescue fluoroscopy" in cases in which ICE imaging alone does not allow safe completion of the procedure. Another aspect is the cost of the procedure, provided both EAM and ICE are used.

SUMMARY

Current experience from several centers suggests that the use of ICE during non-fluoroscopy procedures has many potential benefits. First, it may help to develop operator skills in conventional ablation procedures. Second, it allows safe and reproducible TS puncture without a need for fluoroscopy. Third, it can assist EAM of any relevant chamber of the heart and/or aortic or pulmonary cusps. Fourth, it can localize the tip of the ablation catheter relative to anatomic structures. Fifth, it may visualize the VT substrate in patients with structural heart disease. The most important in the adoption of a non-fluoroscopic approach is the willingness of the operator to change his or her routine. More data are needed to demonstrate other advantages of this strategy: prevention of orthopedic problems and fatigue as a result of wearing X-ray protection apparel.

DISCLOSURES

JK reports personal fees from Biosense Webster, Biotronik, Boston Scientific, Medtronic, Abbott (St Jude Medical), Merit Medical, Daiichi Sankyo, Boehringer Ingelheim, BMS, MSD, Pfizer, Merck, and Bayer for lectures, advisory boards, and consultancy.

JH and FL do not report any potential conflict of interest.

CLINICS CARE POINTS

- Intracardiac echocardiography allows safe and efficacious guidance of non-fluoroscopic catheter ablation procedures.
- Transseptal puncture guided by intracardiac echocardiography is safe and reproducible.
- Non-fluoroscopic electrophysiological procedures decrease radiation burden, both for patients and operators, and may alleviate fatigue of the operators by avoiding the use of lead aprons.

SUPPLEMENTARY DATA

Supplementary data to this article can be found online at https://doi.org/10.1016/j.ccep.2021.03.004.

REFERENCES

1. Klein LW, Miller DL, Balter S, et al. Occupational health hazards in the interventional laboratory: time for a safer environment. Radiology 2009;250(2):538–44.
2. Ozyilmaz I, Ergul Y, Akdeniz C, et al. Catheter ablation of idiopathic ventricular tachycardia in children using the EnSite NavX system with/without fluoroscopy. Cardiol Young 2014;24(5):886–92.
3. Alvarez M, Tercedor L, Herrera N, et al. Cavotricuspid isthmus catheter ablation without the use of fluoroscopy as a first-line treatment. J Cardiovasc Electrophysiol 2011;22(6):656–62.
4. Stec S, Sledz J, Mazij M, et al. Feasibility of implementation of a "simplified, no-X-ray, no-lead apron, two-catheter approach" for ablation of supraventricular arrhythmias in children and adults. J Cardiovasc Electrophysiol 2014;25(8):866–74.
5. Macias R, Uribe I, Tercedor L, et al. A zero-fluoroscopy approach to cavotricuspid isthmus catheter ablation: comparative analysis of two electroanatomical mapping systems. Pacing Clin Electrophysiol 2014;37(8):1029–37.
6. Fernandez-Gomez JM, Morina-Vazquez P, Morales Edel R, et al. Exclusion of fluoroscopy use in catheter ablation procedures: six years of experience at a single center. J Cardiovasc Electrophysiol 2014;25(6):638–44.
7. Ma Y, Qiu J, Yang Y, et al. Catheter ablation of right-sided accessory pathways in adults using the three-dimensional mapping system: a randomized comparison to the conventional approach. PLoS One 2015;10(6):e0128760.
8. Yang L, Sun G, Chen X, et al. Meta-analysis of zero or near-zero fluoroscopy use during ablation of cardiac arrhythmias. Am J Cardiol 2016;118(10):1511–8.
9. Chen G, Wang Y, Proietti R, et al. Zero-fluoroscopy approach for ablation of supraventricular

tachycardia using the Ensite NavX system: a multi-center experience. BMC Cardiovasc Disord 2020; 20(1):48.

10. Ueda A, Soejima K, Miwa Y, et al. MD idiopathic ventricular arrhythmia ablation using non-fluoroscopic catheter visualization system. Int Heart J 2019; 60(1):78–85.

11. Kautzner J, Peichl P. Intracardiac echocardiography in electrophysiology. Herzschrittmacherther Elektrophysiol 2007;18(3):140–6.

12. Luani B, Zrenner B, Basho M, et al. Zero-fluoroscopy cryothermal ablation of atrioventricular nodal reentry tachycardia guided by endovascular and endocardial catheter visualization using intracardiac echocardiography (Ice&ICE Trial). J Cardiovasc Electrophysiol 2018;29(1):160–6.

13. Morton JB, Sanders P, Davidson NC, et al. Phased-array intracardiac echocardiography for defining cavotricuspid isthmus anatomy during radiofrequency ablation of typical atrial flutter. J Cardiovasc Electrophysiol 2003;14(6):591–7.

14. Saad EB, Slater C, Inácio LAC Jr, et al. Catheter ablation for treatment of atrial fibrillation and supraventricular arrhythmias without fluoroscopy use: acute efficacy and safety. Arq Bras Cardiol 2020; 114(6):1015–26.

15. Jan M, Kalinšek TP, Štublar J, et al. Intra-cardiac ultrasound guided approach for catheter ablation of typical right free wall accessory pathways. BMC Cardiovasc Disord 2020;20(1):210.

16. Lamberti F, Di Clemente F, Remoli R, et al. Catheter ablation of idiopathic ventricular tachycardia without the use of fluoroscopy. Int J Cardiol 2015;190:338–43.

17. Baykaner T, Quadros K, Thosani A, et al. Safety and efficacy of zero fluoroscopy transseptal puncture with different approaches. Pacing Clin Electrophysiol 2020;43(1):12–8.

18. Žižek D, Antolič B, Prolič Kalinšek T, et al. Intracardiac echocardiography-guided transseptal puncture for fluoroless catheter ablation of left-sided tachycardias. J Interv Card Electrophysiol 2020. https://doi.org/10.1007/s10840-020-00858.

19. McCauley MD, Patel N, Greenberg SJ, et al. Fluoroscopy-free atrial transseptal puncture. Eur J Arrhythm Electrophysiol 2016;2(2):57–61.

20. Nölker G, Heintze J, Gutleben KJ, et al. Cryoballoon pulmonary vein isolation supported by intracardiac echocardiography: integration of a nonfluoroscopic imaging technique in atrial fibrillation ablation. J Cardiovasc Electrophysiol 2010;21(12):1325–30.

21. Razminia M, Demo H, Arrieta-Garcia C, et al. Non-fluoroscopic ablation of atrial fibrillation using cryoballoon. J Atr Fibrillation 2014;7(1):1093.

22. Kanda T, Masuda M, Kurata N, et al. A saline contrast-enhanced echocardiography-guided approach to cryoballoon ablation. Pacing Clin Electrophysiol 2020; 43(7):664–70. https://doi.org/10.1111/pace.13945.

23. Huang HD, Serafini N, Rodriguez J, et al. Near-zero fluoroscopic approach for laser balloon pulmonary vein isolation ablation: a case study. J Innov Card Rhythm Manage 2020;11(4):4069–74.

24. Reddy VY, Morales G, Ahmed H, et al. Catheter ablation of atrial fibrillation without the use of fluoroscopy. Heart Rhythm 2010;7(11):1644–53.

25. Dello Russo A, Russo E, Fassini G, et al. Role of intracardiac echocardiography in atrial fibrillation ablation. J Atr Fibrillation 2013;5(6):786.

26. Razminia M, Willoughby MC, Demo H, et al. Fluoroless catheter ablation of cardiac arrhythmias: a 5-year experience. Pacing Clin Electrophysiol 2017; 40(4):425–33.

27. Jan M, Žižek D, Kuhelj D, et al. Combined use of electro-anatomic mapping system and intracardiac echocardiography to achieve zero-fluoroscopy catheter ablation for treatment of paroxysmal atrial fibrillation: a single centre experience. Int J Cardiovasc Imaging 2020;36(3):415–22.

28. Ferguson JD, Helms A, Mangrum JM, et al. Catheter ablation of atrial fibrillation Circ. Arrhythm Electrophysiol 2009;2(6):611–9.

29. Bulava A, Hanis J, Eisenberger M. Catheter ablation of atrial fibrillation using zero-fluoroscopy technique: a randomized trial. Pacing Clin Electrophysiol 2015; 38(7):797–809.

30. Stárek Z, Lehar F, Jež J, et al. 3D X-ray imaging methods in support catheter ablations of cardiac arrhythmias. Int J Cardiovasc Imaging 2014;30(7): 1207–23.

31. Rossillo A, Indiani S, Bonso A, et al. J Novel ICE-guided registration strategy for integration of electroanatomical mapping with three-dimensional CT/MR images to guide catheter ablation of atrial fibrillation. J Cardiovasc Electrophysiol 2009;20(4): 374–8.

32. Sadek MM, Ramirez FD, Nery PB, et al. Completely non-fluoroscopic catheter ablation of left atrial arrhyth- mias and ventricular tachycardia. J Cardiovasc Electrophysiol 2019;30(1):78–88.

33. Sánchez JM, Yanics MA, Wilson P, et al. Fluoroless catheter ablation in adults: a single center experience. J Interv Card Electrophysiol 2016;45(2): 199–207.

34. Li MM, Sang CH, Jiang CX, et al. Maternal arrhythmia in structurally normal heart: prevalence and feasibility of catheter ablation without fluoroscopy pacing. Clin Electrophysiol 2019;42(12):1566–72.

35. Drago F, Silvetti MS, Di Pino A, et al. Exclusion of fluoroscopy during ablation treatment of right accessory pathway in children. J Cardiovasc Electrophysiol 2002;13(8):778–82.

36. Smith G, Clark JM. Elimination of fluoroscopy use in a pediatric electrophysiology laboratory utilizing three-dimensional mapping. Pacing Clin Electrophysiol 2007;30(4):510–8.

Intracardiac Echocardiography During Transvenous Lead Extraction

Robert D. Schaller, DO[a],*, Mouhannad M. Sadek, MD[b]

KEYWORDS

- Intracardiac echocardiography • Transvenous lead extraction • Simultaneous traction • Binding
- Avulsion • Flail leaflet

KEY POINTS

- Fluoroscopy is vital to transvenous lead extraction (TLE) but does not provide information related to soft tissues.
- Transesophageal echocardiography is often used during TLE but has limitations.
- Intracardiac echocardiography is used commonly during complex ablation procedures and lends itself to use during TLE.
- Identification of thrombi/vegetation, lead adherence to soft tissues, and complications can aid in TLE procedures.
- Technical improvements, such as increased acutance and three-dimensional functionality, may improve future imaging.

 Video content accompanies this article at http://www.cardiacep.theclinics.com.

INTRODUCTION

Transvenous lead extraction (TLE) is an invaluable procedure within the contemporary management of cardiac implantable electronic devices.[1] Modern tools and techniques render TLE safe and effective, with a similar risk profile to other common procedures within the electrophysiology (EP) landscape.[2,3] Like all invasive procedures, the risks and benefits of TLE must be weighed on a case-by-case basis with consideration of traditional patient-specific variables, such as age, lead type and number, lead dwell time, body mass index, and concomitant comorbidities. Preprocedural chest radiograph is useful in providing the location and number of implanted leads, the course and angulation within the vasculature and heart, and the presence of sternal wires signifying prior cardiac surgery. Similarly, high-quality fluoroscopy is essential to visualize the interaction of the extraction sheaths and leads in real time, and to maintain optimal orientation of the sheath bevel. Although fluoroscopy is adept at visualizing lead components, such as the tip, shocking coils, and conductors, it is poor at visualizing lead insulation or thin, frayed conductors if a lead is lacerated within the body. More importantly, imaging of soft tissue structures on fluoroscopy is limited and typically relegated to shadows. Reliance on fluoroscopic guidance exclusively limits knowledge of vessel narrowing, lead-related thrombi or vegetations, and adherence to the heart or vasculature.

[a] Electrophysiology Section, Division of Cardiovascular Medicine, Perelman School of Medicine at the University of Pennsylvania, Philadelphia, PA, USA; [b] Arrhythmia Service, Division of Cardiology, Department of Medicine, The Ottawa Hospital, Ottawa, Ontario, Canada
* Correspondence:
E-mail address: robert.schaller@pennmedicine.upenn.edu

Card Electrophysiol Clin 13 (2021) 409–418
https://doi.org/10.1016/j.ccep.2021.03.005
1877-9182/21/© 2021 Elsevier Inc. All rights reserved.

COMPLEMENTARY IMAGING MODALITIES
Multidetector Computed Tomography

Multiple advanced imaging modalities are used before and during TLE, each providing complementary information. Preprocedural multidetector computed tomography can identify various degrees of subacute lead perforation, calcific regions, and venous occlusion, and may help stratify procedural risk and guide decision-making.[4–7] Whether a correlation exists between lead-related fibrosis detected on multidetector computed tomography and ease of TLE is the subject of the ongoing Multicenter Imaging in Lead Extraction Study (MILES).[8] Despite this potential utility, lack of real-time imaging and need for additional ionizing radiation limit its value.

Transesophageal Echocardiography

Because availability of echocardiography is a prerequisite for TLE,[1] transesophageal echocardiography (TEE) is convenient and remains the complementary imaging modality of choice in most EP laboratories. The benefits of TEE include a global cardiac view, which is familiar to cardiologists and anesthesiologists. With esophageal placement, there is no concern for sterility or additional venous entry points. However, TEE requires a second operator for real-time monitoring and, because of the size and location of the probe, frequently obscures fluoroscopic visualization of the extraction sheath (**Fig. 1**A). TEE can identify large thrombi and vegetations[9] and acute complications, such as pericardial effusion or tricuspid valve (TV) injury.[10] However, because of the location of the probe posterior to the heart, some regions, including the TV, can prove difficult to reproducibly visualize.[11]

Intravascular Ultrasound

An intravascular ultrasound (IVUS) probe is inserted into the femoral vein, creating cross-sectional, 360-degree views. This can be performed without a second operator, but typically requires the use of a long, precurved sheath because the probe is not deflectable. With excellent near-field vessel visualization, IVUS lends itself to the evaluation of leads within the tubular superior vena cava (SVC).[7] Fibrotic adherences within the heart and vasculature, described as echodense structures along the lead, often highlighted by a linear shadow have also been described.[12] Recently, Beaser and colleagues[13] have shown that intravascular lead adherence correlates with median extraction time and laser pulsations delivered, and another study, the Intravascular Ultrasound Imaging During

Transvenous Lead Extraction (ISEE) trial, is currently enrolling.[14] Despite a long history of IVUS use in the EP laboratory to guide transseptal punctures and monitor for complications, this technology has largely given way to more contemporary ultrasound (US)-based imaging modalities to reliably image other regions within the heart.

Phased-Array Intracardiac Echocardiography

Phased-array intracardiac echocardiography (ICE) has become the dominant advanced imaging modality in the EP laboratory during complex ablation[15] and is an emerging technology in structural interventions[16] because of its three-dimensional bidirectionality, variable frequency, ability to image-remote structures, and rapid identification of complications during a multitude of interventional cardiology procedures.[15] Although ICE does require a separate venous entry point, it can be performed without the need for a second operator. Because of direct visualization of intracardiac structures including leads, ICE has shown an ability to identify thrombi, vegetations, lead "ghosts," and lead-tissue adhesions.[17,18] Herein, we describe the strengths and utility of ICE during TLE.

SET-UP AND WORKFLOW

TLE requires multiple femoral venous access points for fluid resuscitation, femoral snaring, placement of a vascular occlusion balloon, temporary pacing, and ICE. We typically use between two and five venous sheaths depending on the specific scenario. An arterial catheter is placed in the radial artery for invasive blood pressure monitoring with an additional catheter in the femoral artery for possible extracorporeal membrane oxygenation in high-risk patients with a history of previous sternotomy. Two to three left femoral venotomy sites are used to accommodate a wire for a vascular occlusion balloon, ICE, and a temporary pacing catheter if needed. The left side is chosen for ICE because of its proximity to the operator when working at a left-sided chest position and to keep the right side free for snaring.

The patient is prepared and draped to acquire femoral access and perform a baseline ICE study by using a "cummerbund" drape starting at the waistline (**Fig. 2**). The ICE catheter (ViewFlex Xtra, Abbott, Chicago, IL) is placed first to image before placement of other temporary catheters or wires. ICE is guided to the heart using exclusively ICE-guidance and a complete study is performed including visualization of the right atrium (RA), TV, right ventricle (RV), and SVC. Assessment of TV function and identification of baseline pericardial fluid before TLE is essential (**Fig. 3**). Identification

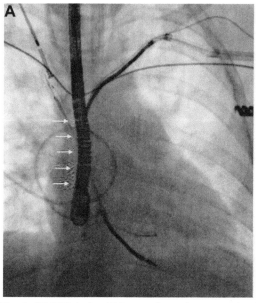
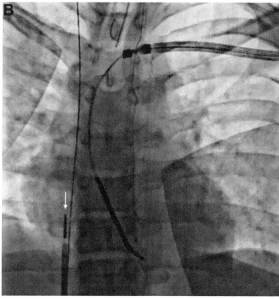

Fig. 1. (A) TEE during TLE. Note how the TEE probe (*yellow arrows*) visually obstructs the region containing the lead in the superior vena cava. (B) Intracardiac echocardiography during TLE. The low-profile probe (*white arrow*) does not visually obstruct the path of the extraction sheath.

of lead-related thrombi or vegetations followed by lead adherences to the vasculature, myocardium, and TV is then performed.

After preoperative ICE assessment is complete, other catheters or wires are placed. The groins are covered by the "cummerbund" sheet to maintain sterility (see **Fig. 2**) and all operators rescrub. ICE is then maneuvered through the sterile sheet allowing for torqueing and advancement and withdrawal of the catheter. If the indication for TLE is infection, the ICE catheter can potentially be handled without the use of a sterile sheet.

LEAD-ADHERENT ECHODENSITIES

Lead-adherent echodensities (LAEs) are classified as thrombi or vegetations and are identified before TLE in three-quarters of patients regardless of anticoagulation status.[19] These masses are typically identified within the RA, just behind or within the TV, but can also be found in the RV and SVC and can have various shapes and sizes (**Fig. 4**, Videos 1 and 2).[20] ICE has been shown to be superior to TEE in identifying LAEs,[17,21] which carry diagnostic and procedural implications, such as

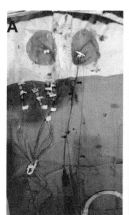
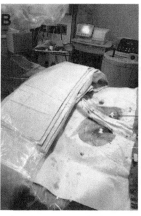
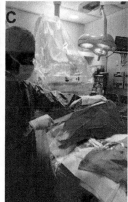
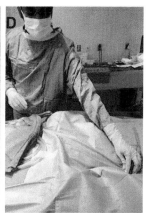

Fig. 2. (A) Femoral venous sheath strategy during transvenous lead extraction. The left-sided sheaths contain a vascular occlusion balloon-compatible wire and the ICE catheter. The right-sided sheaths are left empty for potential snaring. (B) A "cummerbund" sheet is prepared and deployed (C) to maintain sterility after femoral venous access. (D) Further ICE manipulation is performed through the sterile sheet.

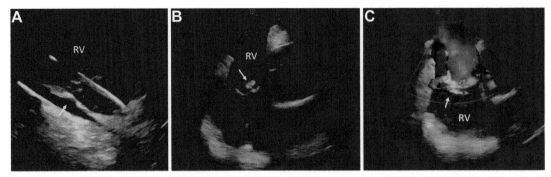

Fig. 3. (*A*) Identification of a baseline pericardial effusion before transvenous lead extraction of a right ventricular lead (*yellow arrow*). (*B*) Flail tricuspid valve leaflet after extraction of a right ventricular lead (*yellow arrow*). (*C*) Eccentric jet of severe tricuspid regurgitation caused by a flail leaflet (*yellow arrow*).

tool selection, and anticipation of complications, such as pulmonary embolism. LAEs identified post-procedurally, frequently because of sheering off of thrombi coating leads, may necessitate postoperative anticoagulation.

Although use of ICE-guided percutaneous tools to prevent embolization of vegetations during TLE has been described,[22] an emerging area of interest is percutaneous aspiration before and after TLE to debulk the LAE (**Fig. 5**).[23,24] Whether this has clinical benefit is not yet known. Lead casts or "ghosts" are also commonly observed in the RV after TLE (see **Fig. 4**H, Video 3), and have been shown to be associated with increased mortality after extraction for infectious purposes.[18] However, attempted removal of such casts is not routinely performed.

VASCULAR ADHESIONS

Vascular injuries, particularly involving the SVC, are dreaded complications and efforts have been made to mitigate this risk by evaluating the tenacity of adhesions before lead removal. The innominate vein is typically not visualized with ICE because of difficulty maneuvering within it, the high likelihood of sheath use in this region regardless of adhesions, and the low rate of injuries to these vessels. The SVC, however, lends itself to evaluation by ICE because of its location and size. Although SVC injuries are rare, they are unpredictable and carry high morbidity and mortality.[25] Ability to identify binding sites here is helpful for procedural planning and risk assessment.

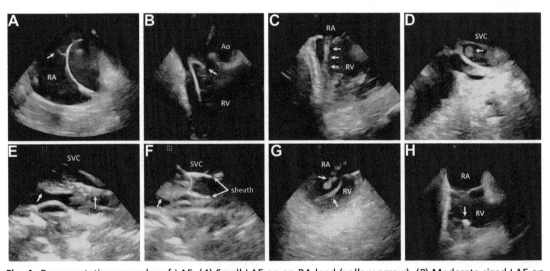

Fig. 4. Representative examples of LAE. (*A*) Small LAE on an RA lead (*yellow arrow*). (*B*) Moderate-sized LAE on an RV lead within the TV (*yellow arrow*). (*C*) Thickened RV lead that is coated with thrombus within the RA and RV (*yellow arrow*). (*D*) Lobulated LAE within the superior vena cava (*yellow arrow*). (*E*) Thrombus (*white arrow*) coating a lead within the SVC. (*F*) An extraction sheath (*dotted line*) approaching and compressing the thrombus within the SVC (*single yellow arrow*). (*G*) Resultant multilobulated thrombus remaining in the RA/RV, presumably sheared off from the extraction process (*yellow arrows*). (*H*) Lead-related "cast" after TLE of an RV lead that showed calcific binding before removal (*yellow arrow*). Ao, aorta.

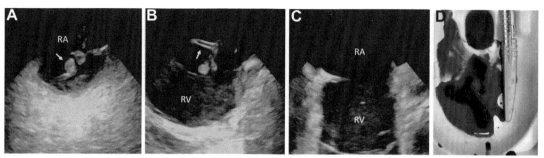

Fig. 5. Attempted aspiration of a thrombus after TLE. (*A*) Multilobulated thrombus in the right atrium (RA) after TLE of an RA lead. (*B*) Thrombus captured by the aspiration sheath. (*C*) Resultant intracardiac echocardiography image after thrombus aspiration, some of which was captured (*D*) and some presumably embolized to the lung.

We have demonstrated that identification of vascular or myocardial adhesions by ICE is associated with a more complex extraction procedure.[19] Leads that show no evidence of adherence (**Fig. 6**A) have a presumably lower risk of SVC injury. It is difficult to distinguish between leads lying on the SVC wall and those that are adhered to the SVC if calcific adhesions are not present (see **Fig. 6**B). Dynamic assessment, using slight traction from above or below, by way of snaring, to assess simultaneous movement of the lead and SVC is more definitive (see **Fig. 6**C, Video 4). Real-time monitoring of the SVC during TLE, however, may not be practical, because traction on the lead frequently causes the lead-tissue interface to leave the imaging plane. However, preprocedural identification of binding sites can aid in risk-stratification and guide extraction technique and tool selection. Additionally, the presence of SVC adhesions may warrant prophylactic placement of a vascular occlusion balloon[19,26] or use of simultaneous countertraction from above and below to increase the separation between the lead and SVC, and create a more parallel relationship of the two.[27] The ability of ICE to identify an SVC laceration above the pericardial reflection, however, is not well established and directing the catheter upward within the SVC during a potential

injury might be contraindicated because it could potentially exacerbate a laceration. However, considering that a presumed SVC injury requires immediate escalation of therapy, including use of an occlusion balloon and urgent surgical intervention, soft tissue imaging in this scenario may have limited value.

RIGHT ATRIUM, TRICUSPID VALVE, AND THE SUBVALVULAR APPARATUS

The RA lead tip can easily be visualized within the RA appendage or free wall, but identifying the degree of binding is challenging because of the thin tissue of the free wall and complex anatomy of the RA appendage. Although significant binding to the eustachian ridge can occasionally be seen (Video 5), which might alter the degree of traction placed on the lead during TLE, ICE imaging of the RA rarely changes management. The TV, however, is highly susceptible to injury and is likely an underrecognized phenomenon because of a lack of dedicated US-based imaging during TLE. In cases where an RV lead pierces the valve,[28] damage is caused by sheaths passing through the valve leaflets. More commonly, lead fibrosis to the TV, subvalvular apparatus, or papillary muscles (see **Figs. 3**B,C, **7**, **8**) can result in valvular

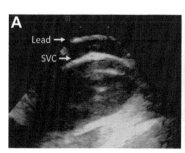
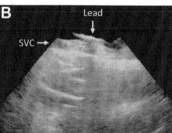
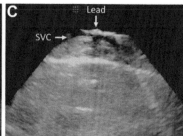

Fig. 6. (*A*) Lead within the SVC with no evidence of adhesions to the wall. (*B*) Lead touching the lateral wall of the SVC. (*C*) Traction on the lead from above pulls the SVC along with it, signifying adherence.

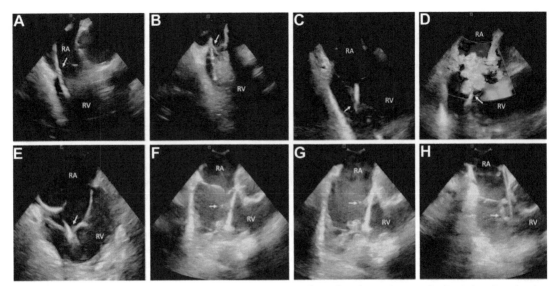

Fig. 7. (*A*) Suggestion of an RV lead adhesion to the TV is confirmed with traction on the lead showing simulta-neous movement of the lead and the TV (*B*). (*C*) An RV lead appears to be adhered to a TV leaflet, supported by a color Doppler jet of tricuspid regurgitation tacking the lead (*D*). (*E*) An RV lead adhered to two TV leaflets. (*F*) Echogenicity of subvalvular tissue suggesting adhesion is confirmed with lead traction showing concomitant movement (*G*). (*H*) Lead cast is seen after successful lead extraction.

damage.[29] In our experience, it is more common to identify lead binding to the subvalvular apparatus including the chordae and papillary muscles (**Fig. 8**), as described in pathologic studies showing intense fibrosis of the implantable cardioverter-defibrillator electrode-myocardial interface.[30] TLE in this setting without concurrent sheath countertraction can result in avulsion in-juries and increased tricuspid regurgitation (see **Figs. 3**B,C, Video 6).

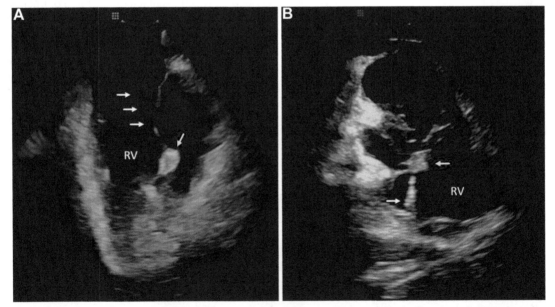

Fig. 8. An RV lead (*white arrows*) adhered to the tricuspid valve papillary muscles (*yellow arrow*). Note the echo-genicity of the papillary muscle at the contact point with the lead, signifying a calcific adhesion (*A*). Gentle trac-tion on the RV lead (*white arrow*) pulls the papillary muscle away from the myocardium, connected only by a thin piece of tissue. This patient was referred for surgical extraction.

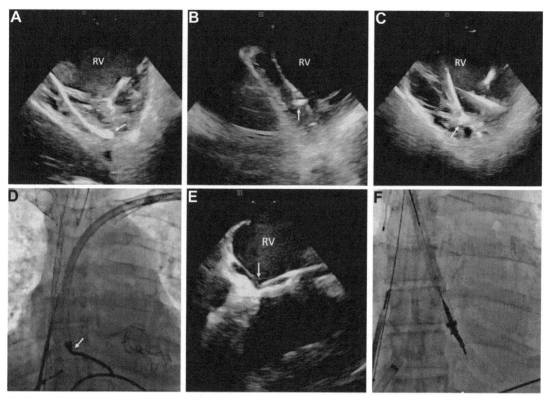

Fig. 9. Lead adhesions to the RV. (*A, B*) Bright echogenic appearance near the lead tip suggests calcific adherence. (*C*) Two RV leads with one showing adhesion to the moderator band–papillary muscle complex (*yellow arrow*) and one free of obvious adhesions. (*D*) Shocking coil adhered to the inferior RV wall creating a suboptimal laser sheath orientation and confirmed with ICE (*E*). Approach from the right internal jugular with a mechanical dissection sheath results in improved sheath orientation and successful lead extraction (*F*).

Because of its proximity to the TV, ICE can identify leaflet adhesions by evaluating for independent movement of the lead and leaflet. The septal leaflet, however, is challenging to visualize, and gentle lead traction may unmask an adhesion (**Figs. 7**F,G, Video 7). Another clue as to lead-valve adhesion is a color Doppler jet that tracks along only the lead (see **Fig. 7**D). Dense, calcific adhesions to the papillary muscles frequently result in enhanced echogenicity of the papillary

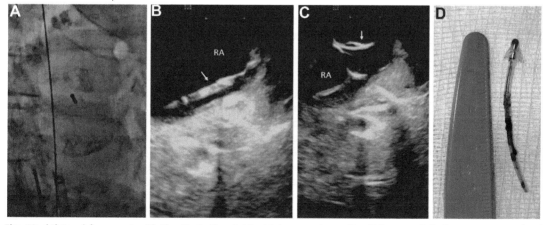

Fig. 10. (*A*) Lead fragment with the tip in the right atrial appendage after it lacerated during transvenous lead extraction. (*B*) ICE suggests the tip includes a long strand of insulation (*yellow arrow*), invisible on fluoroscopy. (*C*) The strand of insulation is snared and removed with a Goose Neck Snare (*yellow arrow*) using ICE-guidance. (*D*) Gross specimen of the lead fragment.

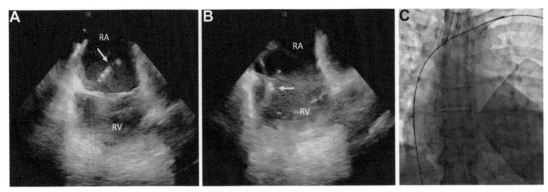

Fig. 11. (*A*) A strand of lead insulation (*yellow arrow*) broken off during transvenous lead extraction within the right atrium and right ventricle causing mechanical arrhythmias. (*B*) The strand has been captured with a Goose Neck Snare (*yellow arrow*) using intracardiac echocardiography-guidance. (*C*) Note how the strand of insulation is not visible before removal using traditional fluoroscopy.

muscle adjacent to the lead (see **Fig. 8**) and gentle traction on the lead from above, resulting in simultaneous movement, can confirm this finding. As opposed to monitoring of the SVC, ICE is steadily positioned in the RA to monitor the TV in real time during TLE (see **Fig. 1**B).

Excessive lead traction during TLE with TV or papillary muscle adhesions can result in TV damage (see **Figs. 3**B,C, Video 6) and this risk is mitigated by monitoring points of adhesion with ICE, to avoid too much traction on the adhered segment. If this is not possible, the lead is snared from below to use simultaneous countertraction and buffer the traction exerted on the bound segment, with the ultimate goal of using the sheath to dissect through the adhesions. The identification of these "vulnerable" valves can aid in dynamic risk assessment, tool selection, and potentially lead to referral for surgical extraction or extraction deferral entirely in elective cases.[31] The degree of tricuspid regurgitation is reassessed post-procedurally to help guide further management in cases where there is a significant change.

RIGHT VENTRICLE

Adhesions within the RV are common because of the thickness of the ventricular myocardium, extensive trabeculations, and frequent presence of a shocking coil (**Fig. 9**, Video 8). The identification of adhesions at the lead tip has been correlated with more challenging TLE procedures (**Figs. 9**A,B).[19] This finding can influence tool selection and extraction strategies including use of mechanical rotational sheaths or approaches from various nontraditional regions to enhance the sheath angle (see **Figs. 9**D,E,F). It is also common to pull the myocardium away from the pericardium when lead traction is applied, creating a

potential space that can give the appearance of pericardial effusion on TEE. ICE can help elucidate this finding as pseudotamponade and avoid unnecessary emergent surgery (Video 9).[32]

SNARING

Lead fragments containing metallic components are typically visible on fluoroscopy. However, those with thin metal components or lead insulation by itself may not be visible, and US-based imaging is helpful to identify and remove them. This is of particular importance when TLE is for lead-related endocarditis (**Fig. 10**) where complete hardware removal is desired, or if the lead fragment has become arrhythmogenic (**Fig. 11**, Video 10). In cases of lead laceration with a lead-fragment interacting with the TV, a decision is made regarding the need for snaring attempts if valvular function is compromised.[29] ICE is helpful to identify these fragments and localize them within the heart or vasculature in real time. Additionally, the sheath tip is used to estimate where the fragment resides fluoroscopically before snaring.[33,34]

SUMMARY

ICE holds unique advantages including high-acutance near-field views of lead and valvular structures, which can aid in risk-stratification before and during TLE. Its use by the modern day electrophysiologist performing TLE is appealing, although there is a learning curve. Further studies regarding ICE-based risk assessment and future technological improvements, including three-dimensionality, may further increase its utility during TLE.

CLINICS CARE POINTS

- ICE imaging is used during a multitude of contemporary cardiac procedures and lends itself to use during TLE.

- Because of operator positioning at the chest and sterility requirements, ICE use by the primary operator has a learning curve.

- Preoperative risk assessment and intraoperative dynamic imaging can alter procedural strategies including choice of tools and techniques.

- ICE is superior to TEE in identifying LAEs, which may have diagnostic and therapeutic implications.

- Injury to the tricuspid valve during TLE might be underreported because of a lack of dedicated US-based imaging, representing an opportunity for future studies based on ICE imaging.

DISCLOSURE

Dr Schaller has served as a consultant for Philips. This study was funded in part by the Koegel Family EP Research Fund.

SUPPLEMENTARY DATA

Supplementary data related to this article can be found online at https://doi.org/10.1016/j.ccep.2021.03.005.

REFERENCES

1. Kusumoto FM, Schoenfeld MH, Wilkoff BL, et al. 2017 HRS expert consensus statement on cardiovascular implantable electronic device lead management and extraction. Heart Rhythm 2017; 14(12):e503–51.

2. Maytin M, Epstein LM, Henrikson CA. Lead extraction is preferred for lead revisions and system upgrades: when less is more. Circ Arrhythm Electrophysiol 2010;3(4):413–24 [discussion 424].

3. Bohnen M, Stevenson WG, Tedrow UB, et al. Incidence and predictors of major complications from contemporary catheter ablation to treat cardiac arrhythmias. Heart Rhythm 2011;8(11):1661–6.

4. Balabanoff C, Gaffney CE, Ghersin E, et al. Radiographic and electrocardiography-gated noncontrast cardiac CT assessment of lead perforation: modality comparison and interobserver agreement. J Cardiovasc Comput Tomogr 2014;8(5):384–90.

5. Ehieli WL, Boll DT, Marin D, et al. Use of preprocedural MDCT for cardiac implantable electric device lead extraction: frequency of findings that change management. AJR Am J Roentgenol 2017;208(4): 770–6.

6. Holm MA, Vatterott PJ, Gaasedelen EN, et al. Algorithm for the analysis of pre-extraction computed tomographic images to evaluate implanted lead-lead interactions and lead-vascular attachments. Heart Rhythm 09 Jan 2020;17(6):1009–16.

7. Vatterott PJ, Syed IS, Khan AH. Lead extraction imaging. Card Electrophysiol Clin 2018;10(4):625–36.

8. Available at: https://clinicaltrials.gov/ct2/show/NCT03772704. Accessed April 6, 2021.

9. Bahadur S, Evans TL, Patel V, et al. Intraoperative transesophageal echocardiography alters surgical plan for laser lead extraction. Anesthesiology 2017; 126(1):164.

10. Strachinaru M, Kievit CM, Yap SC, et al. Multiplane/3D transesophageal echocardiography monitoring to improve the safety and outcome of complex transvenous lead extractions. Echocardiography 2019; 36(5):980–6.

11. Park SJ, Gentry JL 3rd, Varma N, et al. Transvenous extraction of pacemaker and defibrillator leads and the risk of tricuspid valve regurgitation. JACC Clin Electrophysiol 2018;4(11):1421–8.

12. Bongiorni MG, Di Cori A, Soldati E, et al. Intracardiac echocardiography in patients with pacing and defibrillating leads: a feasibility study. Echocardiography 2008;25(6):632–8.

13. Beaser AD, Aziz Z, Besser SA, et al. Characterization of lead adherence using intravascular ultrasound to assess difficulty of transvenous lead extraction. Circ Arrhythm Electrophysiol 2020 Aug; 13(8):e007726.

14. Available at: https://clinicaltrials.gov/ct2/show/NCT04055740. Accessed April 6, 2021.

15. Enriquez A, Saenz LC, Rosso R, et al. Use of intracardiac echocardiography in interventional cardiology: working with the anatomy rather than fighting it. Circulation 2018;137(21):2278–94.

16. Frangieh AH, Alibegovic J, Templin C, et al. Intracardiac versus transesophageal echocardiography for left atrial appendage occlusion with watchman. Catheter Cardiovasc Interv 2017;90(2):331–8.

17. Narducci ML, Pelargonio G, Russo E, et al. Usefulness of intracardiac echocardiography for the diagnosis of cardiovascular implantable electronic device-related endocarditis. J Am Coll Cardiol 2013;61(13):1398–405.

18. Narducci ML, Di Monaco A, Pelargonio G, et al. Presence of 'ghosts' and mortality after transvenous lead extraction. Europace 2017;19(3):432–40.

19. Sadek MM, Cooper JM, Frankel DS, et al. Utility of intracardiac echocardiography during transvenous lead extraction. Heart Rhythm 2017;14(12):1779–85.

20. Caiati C, Pollice P, Lepera ME, et al. Pacemaker lead endocarditis investigated with intracardiac

echocardiography: factors modulating the size of vegetations and larger vegetation embolic risk during lead extraction. Antibiotics (Basel) 2019;8(4): 228.

21. Sadek MM, Cooper JM, Schaller RD. Lead-adherent echodensities: the rule rather than the exception! JACC Clin Electrophysiol 2019;5(7):867.

22. Dello Russo A, Di Stasi C, Pelargonio G, et al. Intracardiac echocardiogram-guided use of a Dormia basket to prevent major vegetation embolism during transvenous lead extraction. Can J Cardiol 2013; 29(11):1532 e1511–1533.

23. Richardson TD, Lugo RM, Crossley GH, et al. Use of a clot aspiration system during transvenous lead extraction. J Cardiovasc Electrophysiol 2020;31(3): 718–22.

24. Rusia A, Shi AJ, Doshi RN. Vacuum-assisted vegetation removal with percutaneous lead extraction: a systematic review of the literature. J Interv Card Electrophysiol 2019;55(2):129–35.

25. Bashir J, Fedoruk LM, Ofiesh J, et al. Classification and surgical repair of injuries sustained during transvenous lead extraction. Circ Arrhythm Electrophysiol 2016;9(9).

26. Wilkoff BL, Kennergren C, Love CJ, et al. Bridge to surgery: best practice protocol derived from early clinical experience with the bridge occlusion balloon. Federated agreement from the Eleventh Annual Lead Management Symposium. Heart Rhythm 2017;14(10):1574–8.

27. Schaller RD, Sadek MM, Cooper JM. Simultaneous lead traction from above and below: a novel technique to reduce the risk of superior vena cava injury during transvenous lead extraction. Heart Rhythm 2018;15(11):1655–63.

28. Wilner BR, Coffey JO, Mitrani R, et al. Perforated tricuspid valve leaflet resulting from defibrillator leads: a review of the literature. J Cardiovasc Surg 2014;29(4):470–2.

29. Schaller RD, Sadek MM, Luebbert JJ, et al. Transjugular lead fragment extraction to improve tricuspid regurgitation. Heartrhythm Case Rep 2015;1(3): 95–8.

30. Epstein AE, Kay GN, Plumb VJ, et al. Gross and microscopic pathological changes associated with nonthoracotomy implantable defibrillator leads. Circulation 1998;98(15):1517–24.

31. Maheshwari A, Desai ND, Giri J, et al. Use of intracardiac echocardiography during transvenous lead extraction to avoid a catastrophic injury. JACC Clin Electrophysiol 2019;5(6):744–5.

32. Sadek MM, Epstein AE, Cheung AT, et al. Pseudotamponade during transvenous lead extraction. Heart Rhythm 2015;12(4):849–50.

33. Mitsopoulos G, Hanna RF, Brejt SZ, et al. Retrieval of a dislodged catheter using combined fluoroscopy and intracardiac echocardiography. Case Rep Radiol 2015;2015:610362.

34. Lee JC, Gallagher R. Extraction of radiolucent fractured wire components using intracardiac ultrasound during pulmonary vein isolation procedure. Heartrhythm Case Rep 2019;5(5):256–9.

Real-Time 3D Intracardiac Echocardiography

Carola Gianni, MD[a],[*], Domenico G. Della Rocca, MD[a], Rodney P. Horton, MD[a], J. David Burkhardt, MD[a], Andrea Natale, MD[a],[b],[c],[d], Amin Al-Ahmad, MD[a]

KEYWORDS

• Intracardiac echocardiography • 3D echocardiography

KEY POINTS

- Traditional bidimensional (2D) ultrasound is dependent on the performing operator's skill and experience. Three-dimensional (3D) ultrasound can overcome this limitation and improve objectivity by providing volumes to accurately display structures with complex anatomy.
- RT-3D ICE improves the visualization of dynamic cardiac structures and their relationship with catheters and devices employed during interventional procedures.
- With continued improvements in transducer technology and miniaturization, the right tradeoff between size, cost, and image quality can be found and this tool can become the standard modality to guide electrophysiologic procedures.

INTRODUCTION

Intracardiac echocardiography (ICE) is an invaluable tool in electrophysiology. Currently, ICE provides real-time bidimensional (2D) ultrasound imaging obtained by phased-array transducers, allowing for RT assessment of cardiac anatomy along with procedure guidance (transseptal puncture, catheter localization, lesion formation) and complications' monitoring (thrombus formation, pericardial effusion).[1] When performing 2D ultrasound, images are obtained in slices and a three-dimensional (3D) image of the scanned region is mentally reconstructed in the mind of the operator, which is key in extracting relevant information. As such, traditional 2D ultrasound is dependent on the performing operator's skill and experience, which might hinder its benefits and reproducibility. 3D ultrasound can overcome this limitation and improve objectivity by providing volumes to accurately display structures with complex anatomy. Initially, 3D imaging was obtained by moving conventional transducers to acquire a sequence of 2D slices, which were then turned into 3D images during a separate reconstruction phase. This process was time consuming, preventing the application of 3D ultrasound in fields where functional, dynamic information is inextricably linked to morphological information. In recent years, advances in electronic and transducer technology have allowed the development and successful implementation of real-time (RT)-3D ultrasound, which is crucial for applications, such as cardiology and guidance of interventional procedures.

RPH, AN, and AAA received honoraria from Siemens; RPH and AN received honoraria from Philips; AAA and AN received honoraria from NuVera.

All the authors share the same contact information as the corresponding author.

Funding: none.

[a] Texas Cardiac Arrhythmia Institute, St. David's Medical Center, Austin, TX, USA; [b] HCA National Medical Director of Cardiac Electrophysiology, Nashville, TN, USA; [c] Interventional Electrophysiology, Scripps Clinic, La Jolla, CA, USA; [d] MetroHealth Medical Center, Case Western Reserve University School of Medicine, Cleveland, OH, USA

* Corresponding author.

E-mail address: carola.gianni@gmail.com

Card Electrophysiol Clin 13 (2021) 419–426
https://doi.org/10.1016/j.ccep.2021.03.006

Herein, we provide an overview of the current ultrasound technologies which allow for RT-3D imaging, with a focus on their application for 3D ICE.

3D ULTRASOUND TECHNOLOGY

The core of 3D imaging is the acquisition and display of volume datasets, as opposed to 2D imaging where tomographic slices are obtained to show of the region of interest. To obtain high-quality full-volume 3D images of dynamic structures in real-time, special ultrasound probes are necessary to acquire raw data, that is, fully-sampled matrix phased-array transducers are necessary.

In basic terms, ultrasound transducers are composed of piezoelectric crystals which convert electric currents into ultrasound waves and generate electric currents in response to their returning echoes to create an image of the region of interest. The timing and strength of such echoes determine the location and composition of the structure reflecting the sound wave, which is displayed as a point on a screen with a set brightness and depth. Traditional linear or curved array transducers are composed of piezoelectric crystals arranged in a single row which fire simultaneously,

creating a planar ultrasound beam (**Fig. 1**). The resulting image has a rectangular or trapezoidal shape (linear or sector field of view), according to the type of transducer. In phased-array transducers, piezoelectric crystals fire sequentially (phasing) in order to direct the sound waves in a specific direction: this electronic steering creates a trapezoidal image (sector field of view) which is wider than the transducer itself (see **Fig. 1**). As such, phased-array transducers are suitable for echocardiography, since the transducer has a small footprint (can fit between the ribs, inside the esophagus, or within the tip of a catheter), but is capable of producing an image that spreads over a wider area with increasing depth.

For traditional 2D imaging, the crystal elements in phased-array transducers are arranged in a single row (linear array) and produce an ultrasound beam that propagates in the axial (or radia; beam depth) and lateral (or azimuth; beam width) direction to produce a tomographic slice (**Fig. 2**). Initially, 3D images were obtained by traditional linear phased-array transducers mechanically moved by an integrated or external motor. The motor guides the transducer to tilt, rotate, or translate in a controlled fashion according to a

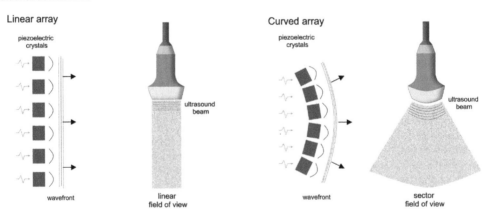

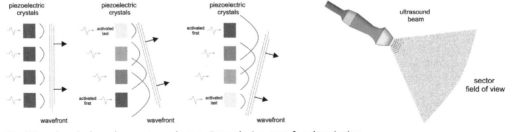

Fig. 1. Traditional and phased-array transducers. See relative text for description.

Spatial resolution

2D sector

3D volume

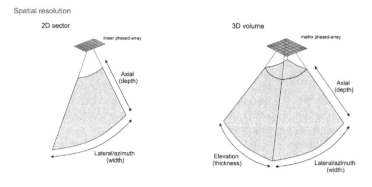

Fig. 2. Linear and matrix phased-array transducers. See relative text for description.

Temporal resolution

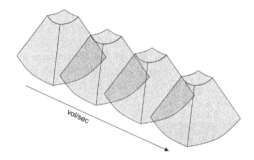

prescribed angle, and volumes are created by combining multiple, regularly-spaced tomographic slices from the traditional array. However, the acquisition of multiple tomographic slices and reconstruction of relative volumes is not immediate, and 3D images obtained by mechanical 3D transducers cannot display dynamic information in real-time.[2] For cardiac applications, a new type transducer has been developed, in which the crystal elements are arranged in rows and columns to form a grid (matrix array).[3] Crystal elements are simultaneously and independently activated (fully-sampled), with phased firing to produce a 3D ultrasound beam that propagates in the axial, lateral, and elevation (slice thickness) direction to produce a pyramidal volume dataset (see **Fig. 2**). A 2D imaging linear phased-array transducer typically contains hundreds of elements, whereas 3D imaging matrix phased-array transducers contain thousands. In 2D linear transducers, each crystal element is connected to the ultrasound machine via a cable constructed from hundreds of small-diameter coaxial wires: this is not possible for 3D matrix transducers, as it would make the cable impractically large. The main breakthrough that has allowed the manufacturing of fully-sampled matrix phased-array transducers used in cardiology is the advent of electronics miniaturization: several circuit boards are integrated into the transducer, where image processing initiates.[3] Signals from each crystal element are summed in the circuit boards reducing the number of coaxial wires composing the cable that connects the transducer to the ultrasound machine.

REAL-TIME 3D IMAGING

Spatial resolution is the ability to distinguish two structures as separate in space and in 3D imaging is comprised of axial, lateral, and elevation resolution (see **Fig. 2**). Axial (depth) resolution, the ability to separate structures parallel to the ultrasound beam, depends on the transducer's frequency and is the same at any point along the beam. By increasing the number of waves traveling within a given distance, higher-frequency waves have a higher axial resolution. However, high-frequency waves are more attenuated because of their shorter wavelength, resulting in a limited depth of penetration. For cardiac ultrasound applications (including 3D ICE, which is mainly used to visualize left-sided structures), more penetration is needed and probes are designed to produce ultrasound waves that range in frequency from 1.5 to 12.0 MHz. Lateral (width) and elevation (thickness) resolution is the ability to separate structures perpendicular to the ultrasound beam and depend on the beam volume, which is a function of the transducer's array design and is affected by the size and depth of volume acquisition: wider, deeper beams diverge further than narrow, shallow beams, decreasing the lateral and elevation resolution.

RT-3D imaging also relies on high temporal resolution (see **Fig. 2**), which is the ability to detect that a structure has moved over time. As with 2D imaging, there is an inverse relationship between temporal resolution (volume frame rate) and spatial resolution (volume field of view), with an increase in one causing a decrease in the other (ie, it takes less time to scan one volume of a narrow field of view). As such, to obtain large field of view (full volume acquisition) images, multi-beat (2–6 beats) gated acquisitions are necessary, which are more difficult to perform.[4] This is because they require absence of patient's motion (including respiration) and a regular heartbeat for the duration of the acquisition to prevent "stitching", an artifact in which sequential volume datasets are not lined up, resulting in a distorted image. To obtain real-time, single-beat, smooth images of cardiac motion (live acquisition), a relatively narrow field of view focused to the region of interest (eg, cardiac valves or left atrial appendage) should be used. This way, RT-3D images can be obtained with sufficient spatial and temporal resolution to guide interventional procedures.

3D images are usually displayed as pyramidal volumetric datasets, which are manipulated during or after image acquisition with cropping and rotation.[5] During image manipulation, surrounding superfluous structures are removed and the viewing perspective is changed to obtain a cut plane that best displays the structure of interest. For example, in case of the left atrial appendage, the interatrial septum and most of the left atrium are cropped off and the appendage is visualized "en face" (**Fig. 3**). Another commonly employed technique to display 3D images is the multiplanar

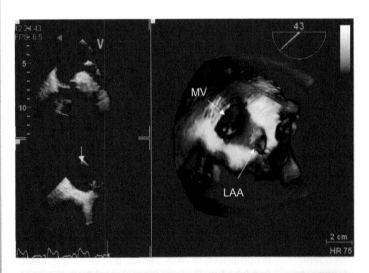

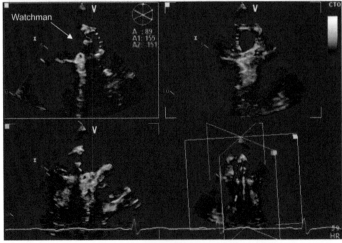

Fig. 3. 3D image display (transesophageal echocardiography). (*Top*) Cropping and rotation of a pyramidal volumetric dataset to display the relationship between the mitral valve (MV) and left atrial appendage (LAA). (*Bottom*) Multiplanar reconstruction of a Watchman device used for LAA occlusion, with simultaneous display of three orthogonal cutting planes (roughly 45°, 90°, 135° views). Images were obtained with the 6VT-D transducer (multifrequency, fully-sampled matrix phased-array) and processed on the Vivid E9 ultrasound machine (GE Vingmed Ultrasound; Horten, Norway).

reconstruction (MPR) mode. In MPR, the volumetric data set is sliced to obtain multiple simultaneous 2D views from different cutting planes. These can be selected from virtually any ultrasound window, so that unique views (impossible to obtain with manipulation of a 2D transducer) can be displayed to better define the anatomical structures of interest. As such, 3D images provide unique sets of information, improving the evaluation of cardiac function and morphology and a more personalized ultrasound guidance for interventional procedures.

3D INTRACARDIAC ECHOCARDIOGRAPHY

Compared to RT-3D transthoracic or transesophageal echocardiography, where spatial and temporal resolution are the main factors affecting probe design, ICE has unique challenges: the probe is a single-use catheter with a restricted diameter (8-Fr to 10-Fr ie, 2.67 to 3.33 mm), which limits the size of transducer and connecting cable. Despite this, spatiotemporal resolution and penetration should still be high to be valuable, while trying to limit the costs of a disposable probe.

3D ICE imaging was pioneered in 2002 at Duke University by the same group who first developed phased-array transducers in the 1970s. The first 3D ICE images were created in animals by using a matrix phased-array transducer operating at 5 MHz within a 12-Fr catheter.[6] While showing good temporal resolution (up to 60 vol/s), spatial resolution was limited by the need to connect each crystal element to the ultrasound machine with separate coaxial wires (miniaturization was still limited): as such, the array could not be operated fully and the active crystal elements were limited to 64, resulting in poor resolution and penetration.

The first in-human 3D ICE images were obtained in 2006 by post-processing a sequence of ECG-gated 2D slices acquired by an ICE catheter (AcuNav; Siemens, Erlangen, Germany) mechanically rotated by an external motor.[7] The AcuNav is a steerable 10F ICE catheter with a linear phased-array multifrequency (5.5 to 10.0 MHz) transducer with 64 crystal elements providing a 90° lateral sector field of view with penetration up to 16 cm. Thus, 3D images obtained with this technique showed adequate depth as well as good axial, lateral, and temporal resolution. However, this type of 3D imaging is not in real-time, with acquisition and reconstruction taking up to 3 to 5 minutes, thus lacking the dynamic aspect which is key for cardiac imaging.

Mirroring the progresses of non-intracardiac ultrasound, in the 2010s different transducer technologies were developed to achieve high-quality 3D-RT imaging. One approach was the use of a micromotor integrated into the ICE catheter which rotates a 6.2 MHz linear phased-array transducer located within the catheter tip. While providing excellent spatial resolution (with a field of view up to 90° lateral × 180° elevation) and adequate penetration, in-vivo testing in animals showed that volume frame rates were too slow to provide smooth cardiac imaging, ranging from 1 vol/s (180° elevation) to 10 vol/s (45° elevation).[8] With miniaturization, a fully-sampled matrix phased-array 10-Fr catheter has been developed, with a field of view of up to 90° lateral × 90° elevation and a frame rate of 30 vol/s. This device was tested in animals, proving to be able to provide adequate anatomic and functional cardiac imaging.[9] An alternate approach is the use of a traditional linear phased-array with an helical twist of the face, in which crystal elements are arranged

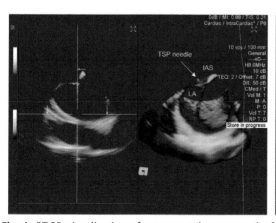 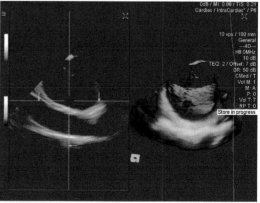

Fig. 4. RT-3D visualization of a transeptal puncture. (*Left*) Tenting of the interatrial septum (IAS) while pushing the transeptal (TSP) needle. (*Right*) Left atrial (LA) access. Images were obtained with the AcuNav Volume transducer positioned in the right atrium and processed on the SC2000 ultrasound machine (Siemens).

in a single row gradually transitioning in their orientation to scan along different planes.[10–12] This design allows to obtain volumes with a field of view of 90° lateral × up to 24° in elevation. This is the technology employed by the only commercially available RT-RD ICE catheter to date, the AcuNav V (Siemens).

AcuNav V AND AcuNav Volume

The AcuNav V ICE catheter uses a helical linear phased-array multifrequency (5.0 to 10.0 MHz) transducer with multiple crystal elements mounted inside the tip of a steerable 10-Fr catheter. As with AcuNav, AcuNav V is steerable in four directions (up to 160°) across two orthogonal planes. This catheter has been successfully used in a wide variety of interventional procedures, ranging from electrophysiology to cardiac structural interventions, including atrial fibrillation ablation, closure of patent foramen ovalis or atrial/ventricular septal defects, balloon valvuloplasty,

transcatheter aortic valve implantation or mitral valve repair, and left atrial appendage occlusion.[13–19] RT-3D images obtained with the AcuNav V catheter have a high frame rate (approximately between 20 and 50 vol/s, based on the volume size), but a relatively small field of view (up to 90° lateral by 24° elevation), which limits its ability to provide a comprehensive visualization of structures of interest, such as the heart valves, pulmonary vein antra, or closure devices.

The new generation, AcuNav Volume, is a 12.5-Fr steerable ICE catheter using the same type of transducer technology, with a longer helical linear phased-array, a greater number of crystal elements, and a higher angular twist-rate. As such, AcuNav V allows to obtain volumetric images with a wider angle (50°) azimuthal elevation and a maximum achievable frame rate of 14 to 20 vol/s.[20] To date, AcuNav Volume has been successfully employed to guide left atrial appendage occlusion procedures.[21,22] In our center, we have

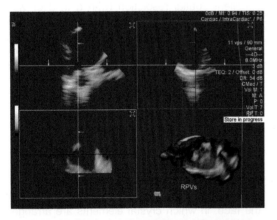

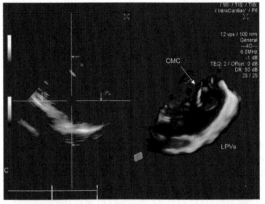

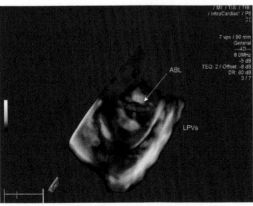

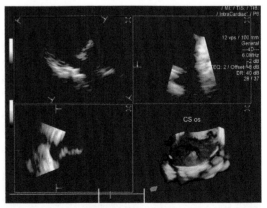

Fig. 5. RT-3D visualization of relevant atrial structures. (*Top left*) Right pulmonary veins (RPVs) antra. (*Top right*) Left pulmonary veins (LVPs) antra showing the circular mapping catheter (CMC) positioned in the left inferior pulmonary vein. (*Bottom left*) Ablation catheter (ABL) positioned on the ridge, anterior to the left inferior pulmonary vein. (*Bottom right*) Coronary sinus (CS) os. Images were obtained with the AcuNav Volume transducer positioned in the right atrium and processed on the SC2000 ultrasound machine.

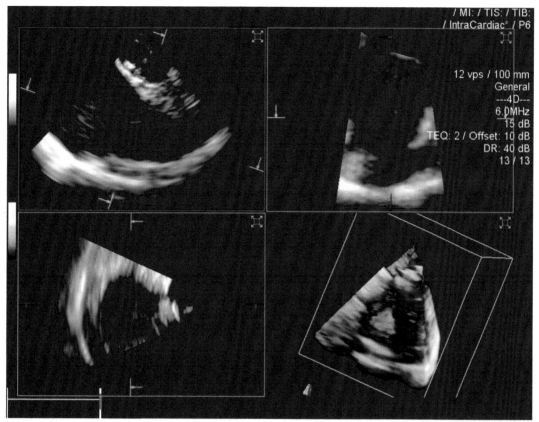

Fig. 6. RT-3D visualization of the left atrial appendage. Multiplanar reconstruction and volumetric rendering of the left arial appendage. Images were obtained with the AcuNav Volume transducer positioned in the right ventricular outflow tract and processed on the SC2000 ultrasound machine.

also tested the AcuNav Volume catheter during atrial fibrillation ablation procedures (see **Figs. 4–6** with relative description), which proved the feasibility of using this catheter to obtain adequate visualization of relevant structures with fairly simple image acquisition and processing.[23]

FUTURE DEVELOPMENTS

To our knowledge, two additional 3D ICE catheters are under development for clinical use and awaiting FDA clearance/CE approval: the 9-Fr steerable VeriSight Pro (Philips; Eindhoven, Netherlands) catheter and the 10-Fr steerable NuVision (NuVera; Los Gatos, CA) catheter. Both use fully-sampled matrix phased-array transducers with hundreds of crystal elements, which allow to acquire volumes with a wider field of view (up to 90° lateral × 90° elevation) and high spatiotemporal resolution. In addition, the NuVision ICE utilizes a novel catheter manipulation design in which a dedicated knob allows to independently rotate the transducer inside the catheter by full 360°. This simplifies image acquisition by reducing

the number and complexity of catheter maneuvers necessary to obtain specific views of the structures of interest.

CONCLUSIONS

RT-3D ICE improves the visualization of dynamic cardiac structures and their relationship with catheters and devices employed during interventional procedures. With continued improvements in transducer technology and miniaturization, the right tradeoff among size, cost, and image quality can be found and this tool can become the standard modality to guide electrophisiological procedures.

CLINICS CARE POINTS

- Three-dimensional (3D) ultrasound reduce operator-dependence by providing volumes to accurately display structures with complex anatomy.
- Real-time 3D intracardiac echocardiography (ICE) allows to visualize cardiac structures in

motion, as well as their relationship with catheter and devices used during interventional procedures.

- During transseptal puncture, 3D ICE can display the full fossa ovalis and simplifies site-selective catheterization to access a specific location in the left atrium (i.e. posterior for pulmonary vein isolation, anterior for ventricular tachycardia ablation, low for left atrial appendage closure) which is key to facilitate many interventional procedures.
- In percutaneous left atrial appendage occlusion procedures, 3D ICE can be an alternative to 3D TEE to determine device sizing and assess closure obviating the need for a second operator.

REFERENCES

1. Enriquez A, Saenz LC, Rosso R, et al. Use of intracardiac echocardiography in interventional cardiology: working with the anatomy rather than fighting it. Circulation 2018;137(21):2278–94.
2. Szabo TL, Lewin PA. Ultrasound transducer selection in clinical imaging practice. J Ultrasound Med 2013;32(4):573–82.
3. Savord B, Solomon R. Fully sampled matrix transducer for real time 3D ultrasonic imaging. In: IEEE symposium on ultrasonics, 2003 [Internet]. Honolulu, HI, USA: IEEE; 2003. p. 945–53. Available at: http://ieeexplore.ieee.org/document/1293556/. Accessed September 1, 2020.
4. Rong LQ. An update on intraoperative three-dimensional transesophageal echocardiography. J Thorac Dis 2017;9(S4):S271–82.
5. Vegas A. Three-dimensional transesophageal echocardiography: principles and clinical applications. Ann Card Anaesth 2016;19(5):35.
6. Smith SW, Light ED, Idriss SF, et al. Feasibility study of real-time three-dimensional intracardiac echocardiography for guidance of interventional electrophysiology. Pacing Clin Electrophysiol 2002;25(3):351–7.
7. Knackstedt C, Franke A, Mischke K, et al. Semiautomated 3-dimensional intracardiac echocardiography: development and initial clinical experience of a new system to guide ablation procedures. Heart Rhythm 2006;3(12):1453–9.
8. Lee W, Griffin W, Wildes D, Buckley D, Topka T, Chodakauskas T, et al. A 10 Fr ultrasound catheter with integrated micromotor for 4D intracardiac echocardiography. 2010 IEEE Int Ultrason Symp. 2010 Oct;833–6.
9. Wildes D, Lee W, Haider B, et al. 4-D ICE: a 2-D array transducer with integrated ASIC in a 10-Fr catheter for real-time 3-D intracardiac echocardiography. IEEE Trans Ultrason Ferroelectr Freq Control 2016;63(12):2159–73.
10. Garbini LJ, Wilser WT. Multi-twisted acoustic array for medical ultrasound 2012. Washington, DC. US 8,206,305 B2.
11. Garbini LJ, Wilser WT. Helical acoustic array for medical ultrasound 2013. Washington, DC. US 9,261,595 B2.
12. Wilser WT, Barnes SR, Garbini LJ. Acoustic array with a shape alloy for medical ultrasound 2016. Washington, DC. US 8,449,467 B2.
13. Fontes-Carvalho R, Sampaio F, Ribeiro J, et al. Three-dimensional intracardiac echocardiography: a new promising imaging modality to potentially guide cardiovascular interventions. Eur Heart J Cardiovasc Imaging 2013;14(10):1028.
14. Brysiewicz N, Mitiku T, Haleem K, et al. 3D real-time intracardiac echocardiographic visualization of atrial structures relevant to atrial fibrillation ablation. JACC Cardiovasc Imaging 2014;7(1):97–100.
15. Silvestry FE, Kadakia MB, Willhide J, et al. Initial experience with a novel real-time three-dimensional intracardiac ultrasound system to guide percutaneous cardiac structural interventions: a phase 1 feasibility study of volume intracardiac echocardiography in the assessment of patients with structural heart disease undergoing percutaneous transcatheter therapy. J Am Soc Echocardiogr 2014;27(9):978–83.
16. Maini B. Real-time three-dimensional intracardiac echocardiography: an early single-center experience. J Invasive Cardiol 2015;27(1):E5–12.
17. Kadakia MB, Silvestry FE, Herrmann HC. Intracardiac echocardiography-guided transcatheter aortic valve replacement: ICE-Guided TAVR. Catheter Cardiovasc Interv 2015;85(3):497–501.
18. Rendon A, Hamid T, Kanaganayagam G, et al. Annular sizing using real-time three-dimensional intracardiac echocardiography-guided trans-catheter aortic valve replacement. Open Heart 2016;3(1):e000316.
19. Patzelt J, Schreieck J, Camus E, et al. Percutaneous mitral valve edge-to-edge repair using volume intracardiac echocardiography: first in human experience. CASE 2017;1(1):41–3.
20. Yastrebov K, Brunel L, Paterson HS, et al. Three-dimensional intracardiac echocardiography and pulmonary embolism. Cardiovasc Ultrasound 2020;18(1):36.
21. Ribeiro J, Braga P, Gama V. New catheter, wide angle imaging, 3D intracardiac echocardiography. Rev Esp Cardiol Engl Ed 2018;71(4):293.
22. Khalili H, Patton M, Taii HA, et al. 4D volume intracardiac echocardiography for intraprocedural guidance of transcatheter left atrial appendage closure. J Atr Fibrillation 2019;12(4):2200.
23. Al-Ahmad A, Camus E, Gianni C, et al. Second generation real-time 3D intracardiac echocardiography for ablation procedures. Heart Rhythm 2017;14(Suppl 5):S229.

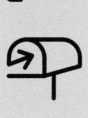